YOGA For Backache Relief

YOGA For Backache Relief

Bharat Thakur

wisdom tree

First published 2005
Reprinted in 2006, 2007, 2008, 2009, 2010, 2011, 2012

ISBN 978-81-8328-006-8

Published by

Wisdom Tree
4779/23, Ansari Road
Darya Ganj, Delhi-110002
Ph. 23247966/67/68

Printed in India

Contents

1

Introduction to Yoga

Patanjali has defined *asana* as *'sthiram sukham asana'* which literally means, stability, a feeling of well-being. *Asanas* or postures are not yoga but they are one of the most important aspects. The science of *asana* can be used in different ways. It can help a man to get rid of disease or remove stress. But yoga is not for disease curing or stress relief. It is a process that can change a man's way of life, though it can be used to cure man of arthritis, back pain or frozen shoulder. This science which was developed by Indian masters over hundreds of years ago works on all aspects of life. It throws light on the philosophical aspect of life and through experimentation provides answers to questions relating to man's existence, like 'Who am I?', 'Where have I come from?', 'What should I do?' etc. Yoga is a beautiful amalgamation. It is a physical science that can give man good health, physical well-being and freedom from disease. It is also a mental science that relaxes, reduces stress, understands the mechanism of the mind and gives mental stability. It knows the art of marrying the physical with the mental body to attain the metaphysical or spiritual body.

Like any other disease, I consider back pain to be a disease because back pain makes a person go from a state of ease to a state of 'dis-ease'. It disturbs the day-to-day function of a man. Backache is inter-linked to all aspects of the human being — the emotional body, fear body, mental body, and stress body. Backache results not only from bad posture, physical injury or bad habits, but also gets accentuated due to a man's mental condition. A stressful man will have a tendency to develop backache. A tired man may also develop back pain. Whatsoever a man experiences at the emotional and mental levels has an effect on the muscles of the body. Stress is known to create muscular contractions and mild spasms, which may get aggravated with bad habits or lifestyle. So the whole process of yoga relaxes, strengthens and cures the root cause of the disease.

We have two brains in the body. In layman's terms, one is the higher brain and the other, the lower. In scientific language, they are the CNS (central nervous system) and the PNS (peripheral nervous system). The higher brain consists of the cerebellum, the cortex, the medulla oblongata, etc. The lower brain consists of the spine, which has 32 pairs of peripheral nerves. These peripheral nerves are spread over the body like an electric circuit regulating all the reflex functions. So the spine must be protected in every possible way because it performs many more functions than the brain. The brain is the decision-maker; the spine is the controller. The philosophy of yoga speaks about a flexible back leading to a slowing down of the aging process. A straight spine is also used for meditative purposes. The final goal of meditation is *samadhi* which is nothing but a union of the three *nadis* (electrical wiring). The left nostril symbolises the *ida nadi,* the right symbolises the *pingala nadi* and in the spine is the most important— the *sushmna nadi.* An important aspect of meditation is to connect the three together. This is called *kundalini* yoga. So maintaining the health of the back, which is directly related to the condition of the spine is important in maintaining the total functionality of the back in day-to-day life and also for reaching higher levels of meditation. Every single posture in yoga has some influence on the back. Practising the *asanas* prescribed in this book will work intensely to relax, strengthen and give your back the freedom of movement that it was designed to have.

2

Understanding Your Back

The spinal column is one of the most amazingly designed structures in Nature. It forms the centre-piece of the human body, providing strength and stability which allow man to walk upright (unique in the animal kingdom), while also offering a wide range of movement to the body in motion.

The spinal column is composed of two elements — the visible vertebral column composed of the vertebrae, and the spinal cord that is enclosed and protected and is made up of nerves.

Backbone (the structural core)

The vertebral column or backbone, extends from the base of the brain to the base of the pelvis. It is made up of 33 separate bones called *vertebrae* which are intricately placed, one on top of the other, and bound together by strong ligaments and spinal joints to provide both stability and flexibility to the human frame. In between the vertebrae are flexible intervertebral discs, which act as shock absorbers, ensuring we safely enjoy the simplest of functions like walking, jumping or riding a bike.

The spinal column is divided into five regions:

Cervical: comprises of the seven topmost vertebrae. This covers the neck region and is responsible for the movement of the head. It is the most flexible part of the spine and hence most prone to injury and pain, like in cervical spondylitis.

Thoracic: comprises of twelve vertebrae. These twelve vertebrae bear indentations for the twelve pairs of ribs to be attached. Together with the ribs and the sternum (breastbone), the vertebrae form a thoracic cage that protects the internal organs. You can feel this thoracic cage move up and down as you breathe in and out.

Lumbar: comprises of five vertebrae. The lumbar region is called the powerhouse of the spine, as it supports the load of the torso. Hence they develop into larger and stronger vertebrae.

Sacrum: comprises of five fused vertebrae. The sacrum, along with the two hip bones and coccyx, form the pelvic girdle (pelvis), which links the torso and the lower limbs. It supports your weight when sitting and standing.

Coccyx: comprises of four fused vertebrae, although the first may be a separate piece. The coccyx forms the very base of the spine and is also referred to as the *tailbone.*

Keeping the vertebral column intact

All the vertebrae of the spine need to be held together strongly and yet in a manner as to allow flexibility of the torso. For this, three separate kinds of joints are employed:

- the *intervertebral discs*, positioned between two adjacent vertebrae form the first joint. Apart from acting as a shock absorber, they make movement in the vertebral column possible.
- the entire vertebral column is bonded by two long *ligaments* — *anterior longitudinal ligament*, attached to the front of the vertebral bodies and which protect the vertebral column against excessive backward bending; *posterior longitudinal ligament*, attached to the back of the vertebral bodies and prevents excessive separation of vertebral bodies while bending forward.
- the third kind of joint is the *facet joint* which prevents the intervertebral joints from being twisted too much or displaced forward.

The rupturing or displacement of any of these joints usually results in what is known as slipped disc.

Spinal cord (information super-highway)

The spinal cord is a collection of nerves that arise in the brain and extend downwards, enclosed and protected within the vertebral column.

Today we know that the nervous system is the most important control system of the body. It has two components — the *central* and the *peripheral nervous systems.*

The central nervous system comprises the brain and spinal cord, while the peripheral nervous system comprises the peripheral nerves, the innervating muscles and organs.

Let us understand the role of the spinal cord. Information passes from the brain, which is the seat of control, through the spinal cord to the various organs and glands. The information is of two types: one passing through somatic nerves whose job is to stimulate the muscles to produce movement (voluntary), and the other through autonomic nerves which control the involuntary functions of different organs, such as the heartbeat. The other kind of information flow is sensory information of the outside world, which passes from the peripheral nerves spread throughout the body through the spinal cord, upwards to the brain. The spinal cord thus functions as an information super-highway for information between the brain and the rest of the organism. In fact, lesions in the spinal cord could produce paralysis in the body below the site of the lesion as nerve transmission is broken from that point onwards. Hence the spinal cord requires protection by the bony segment of the spinal column. It would be very vulnerable otherwise.

The spinal cord is enclosed in the spinal column and passes through the canals of the vertebrae. It is about 45 cm long and extends from the brain stem to the lumbar sacral region of the lower back. The 31 pairs of peripheral spinal nerves originate from the space between adjacent vertebrae in the spinal column, connecting it to the rest of the organism. Some of them are so long that they extend from the spinal cord to the tip of the toe.

These nerves are responsible for conveying all the messages in the peripheral nervous system. They form the body's communication system without the proper functioning of which the body would become a mere vegetable.

S-curve of the spine

In the normal standing posture, the lumbar spine has a natural concave curve or S-shape, known as *lumbar lordosis*. This curvature of the lumbar region is fundamental in providing strength and maintaining the spine's flexibility. In fact this S-curve, along with the skeletal muscles in the back, is responsible for keeping the body upright.

However, through years of sitting, standing and lying down in faulty postures, we gradually lose the S-curvature of the spine and this manifests in a range of spinal problems from backaches to slipped disc, sciatica and others.

Muscles of the back

It would be ridiculous to talk about the spinal column without mentioning the role of the muscles. For, without the muscles the skeleton is really just a heap of bones. The muscles provide movement to the body. There are more than 600 muscles in the human body, most of which are skeletal muscles. That is, they are inserted through muscle tendons at key points in the bones making movement possible and protecting the skeleton.

Along with the spinal column, the muscles located in the back region are fundamental to keeping the torso upright, and in providing movement. Although there are innumerable muscles in different layers protecting the spine, the three most crucial muscles are:

- *Erector spinae,* located behind the abdomen in the lower spine. This small muscle is largely concerned with keeping the body upright.
- *Latissimus dorsi* runs from the lower chest to the lumbar region. Popularly referred to as *lats,* they are responsible for lowering the arms downwards and pulling the body upwards.
- *Trapezius* runs down the back of the neck and along the shoulders. It is the muscle where most of the stress in the body accumulates. That's why you feel tremendously relieved when this muscle is massaged. It is responsible for performing the 'shrugging action', moving the shoulders towards the ears.

As we have seen, the back is an amazing structure, with the spine at the core and the muscles around it to give the back the flexibility and movement it needs in day-to-day life. Practicing yoga on a regular basis will keep the muscles and ligaments strong and flexible, allowing your spinal cord to remain protected and safe from damage.

3

Causes of Backache

Backaches are a result of a combination of reasons — physical, emotional, and mental. Our sedentary lifestyle has definitely contributed to it. So has stress, which is a modern-day affliction. A bad posture, too, is linked to a human being's emotional state. A happy man does not slouch. He walks straight. The psychological and physical make-up of a person are both responsible for this disease. More people suffer from backache than any other form of pain or injury. Yet there are few solutions available. The common understanding is that if you have backache, you have to learn to live with it. And since we are continuously using our backs throughout the day, it becomes difficult to know exactly what triggers the backache and then correct that problem. Though backaches can stem from serious injury, most of the time it is the day-to-day activities, physical and mental, that gradually weaken and ultimately damage the back.

Faulty posture

Bad posture is one of the foremost causes of backache. Through years of misuse, the back takes on a permanent deformity that leads to severe backaches and spasms. This makes it vital to watch your posture while performing even the most innocuous of tasks.

- **Standing:** Always stand straight with the shoulders pushed back slightly; avoid slouching. Also check to see if your weight is equally balanced on both legs.
- **Sitting:** If you have a desk-job, you know how painful it is to sit for a few hours continuously. Choose a chair that is ergonomically designed and that can be adjusted for your height. Always ensure that you get up from your chair every hour and stretch yourself. Move your neck around, stretch your hands upwards, stretch and twist your spine, move your hips, move your feet and stretch your legs. It makes sense to walk a few paces for the body to relieve stiffness.
- **Sleeping:** If you regularly wake up with a bad back, chances are that you are sleeping in a posture that is causing you pain. Try out a new posture to sleep in. Avoid sleeping on your stomach. Also it could be that your mattress and pillow need to be changed. Look for a firm yet supportive mattress.
- **Couch potato:** Everyone loves to laze around on the couch watching TV. Remember that it is destroying your back. Always sit upright and comfortably while watching TV. Avoid slouching or lying down, because chances are that you are straining your neck and back to catch a glimpse of the action.

- **Picking-up things:** Tremendous care must be taken while picking up things off the floor. Most commonly while picking up a bucket of water, or any other load, ensure that you bend your knees and lift the load using your legs, rather than using the muscles of your back.
- **Wrong walking:** A faulty technique of walking will cause tremendous back pain. Always keep your torso upright and your abdominal muscles pulled in while walking. Move your hands and look to power your strides with the muscles in your hips along with the legs.

Driving and travelling

Travel means spending hours stuck behind the wheel of a car or in a bus, train or aircraft. Even if you travel in a comfortable car or fly first-class, travelling can be very difficult. However, small practices can make the journey a lot more comfortable and enjoyable.

- Keep your feet squarely on the floor with your knees slightly higher than your hips for good blood flow.
- Keep your hips and butt squarely against the seat, but curve the lower back, using a pillow or blanket, if necessary.
- Keep your shoulders against the seat with your head directly above and resting against — not above — the headrest.
- Drive with your hands on the sides of the steering wheel, not on the top or bottom.

- Always use your seat belt; it helps support your back.
- When driving, change your visual focal point often.
- Avoid staying still for long; do a few simple exercises every half hour: curl and uncurl your fingers and toes; tighten and then loosen calf, thigh, shoulder and bicep muscles; move your chest as high upwards as possible while pushing out your stomach and pulling your shoulders back.
- Practise a few simple *pranayama* exercises.
- When you are driving and get tired, pull over and take a break or let someone else drive.

Sports and exercise injury

Most sports apply a tremendous strain on the back because of the movement that they involve. Although playing sports strengthens the back, it also places the back in danger very often. Anything can go wrong and you can damage your back very severely. And it need not be just a high contact sport; even a game like golf can do some very serious damage to the spine, either by accident or if you are not careful.

- Playing without warming up puts the body and back in real danger of sustaining serious injury. This applies to any form of exercise; it is essential for the body to be heated before the muscles can be stretched.
- Using the right pair of shoes is extremely important while

walking or running. Choose a pair that provides enough support and cushioning to the foot and ankle, and is light to walk in.

- People very often damage their backs through faulty weight training or overloading in the gym. In the mad rush to increase your muscle mass overnight, you end up trying to lift too heavy a load and obviously damage your back.
- Another common back injury in the gym is caused because you tend to work a lot on the abs while nearly neglecting the back. This one-sided, asymmetrical approach causes strain or injury to your back.

Postnatal care

After the considerable weight that you have been carrying through the previous nine months, the last thing you need is to strain your back while carrying your baby.

At first, new mothers will be lifting 3 to 5 kgs at least 50 times a day. By 12 months they will be chasing and lifting a 8.5 kg child. Two years later, mothers will be lifting a 12 to 15 kg child.

The most difficult part of this lifting is that you often get into an awkward position while lifting the baby from the crib, floor or car seat. It is very easy to develop chronic back pain and pull back muscles while doing this. Hence, it becomes essential to practice proper body mechanics while lifting. This means that you always carry the baby close to your body. While lifting a child up from the floor, bend at your knees, not at your waist, then squat down, tighten your stomach muscles and lift the baby using your leg muscles.

Here are some basic tips to remember:

- Start practising yoga soon after delivery. Ten minutes of stretching exercises each day will restore hip and back flexibility.
- Try to get back to your normal weight within six weeks after giving birth.
- Consider using a front pack to carry the baby when you're walking.
- Don't carry a child on your hip; this strains the back muscles.
- To avoid upper back pain from breast-feeding, bring the baby to your breast; don't bend over to the baby. And sit in an upright chair rather than on a soft couch.

Obesity

Obese and overweight people are more prone to backaches. This is because their girth round the stomach area becomes a tremendous load for the spine to support. We saw that the spine has a natural S-curve, especially prominent in the lumbar region. As a person puts on more weight, the spine loses its natural curvature to compensate for the forward bulge of the stomach. This applies a tremendous strain on both the structure and functioning of the spine. Overweight people complain of terrible back pains. It could also lead to more serious back conditions if you continue to add weight. You do not have to be severely obese; even being slightly overweight strains the back. Try to lose weight and bring your body back to shape — it will bring great relief to your spine.

Stress

The biggest cause of back pain is imbalance in the muscles. This is caused mainly through stress, since stress causes the muscles of one area to tighten, while the muscles on the other side of the back may remain loose. This directly causes muscle pulls and spasms in the back. Also this kind of backache is long-lasting since it has a psycho-somatic (mind-body) root. Hence you need to address the stress before you can cure your backache. Lack of rest, which usually accompanies stress, also causes backache. The body needs its rest period to rejuvenate and heal itself. Every time you deprive it of adequate rest, you will experience some form of discomfort or the other. Stress affects first the peripheral and then the central nervous system in the spine and brain; through yoga you improve the flexibility and mobility of the spine, thereby preventing stress from reaching the higher centres of the brain.

These are the primary causes of backache, and you will surely identify some of them that have troubled you at some stage. Also sometimes, a childhood injury could effect the present condition of your back adversely. Women who wear high heels for long periods are also prone to backaches.

Practising yoga daily goes a long way in dealing with a bad back, both before you damage it and as a therapy once you have injured it. This happens because yoga is unique in that it understands the need of having a strong back, and most of the work emphasises on strengthening and making the back more flexible.

4

Developing a Preventive Lifestyle

Modern day man leads a life that is fundamentally imbalanced. He does little or no physical work. Most of the time is spent in a chair. Speed has become a way of life and things are getting only faster and faster. Man is caught in a rat race and along the way he has forgotten that unless the body is taken good care of, he can never get ahead in this race. Human psychology is such that until a problem arises, we do not pay attention to something. Whether it is our body or car or computer, unless it breaks down, we take it for granted. In the case of machines, the price we pay might be small. But with our body, we pay a huge price. Can you put a price on a backache? How much would you be willing to spend for a cure? A man suffering from a severe backache would say — any amount. Because no amount of money is large enough to get back freedom in the body. Hence, a preventive lifestyle is the singlemost important thing for every human being. It can save you the agony of this painful disease, and it can give you a healthy back for the rest of your life, even if you suffer from no back pain right now.

We saw that most of the spinal injuries arise from a complete lack of awareness while performing some of the most basic daily activities. For instance, a common injury happens while lifting a bucket. And you know how unfocused and unaware you are while doing this. Similarly, watching TV while lounging around or slouching while driving happens only because you are not paying attention while performing these activities. Just recall how often have you suddenly become aware and corrected your posture? However, most of the time people are so wrapped in their thoughts that they neglect their bodies. It is during these lapses really that the worst abuse happens to your body.

In fact the back takes the maximum brunt of your 'absence'. Unconsciously your posture gets affected by your thoughts and emotions. Let us consider depression. You can immediately tell if a person is feeling low and depressed without even knowing him. We do this by simply looking at him, and his body tells us. The tell-tale signs of a depressed person are the drooping of the shoulders, slouching of the back and drooping of the head. And he is always caught up in some self-occupying thought process. On the contrary, observe a happy man. He always has his back straight and shoulders pushed back. And he is very much present. The mind-body connection here becomes very transparent. If depression makes the back and shoulders slouch, then by keeping the back straight, can we stay out of depression? Strange as it may seem, this is true. *Yogis* have researched on the body and mind in great depth, and one of the innumerable insights to come out of this research is that as long as the back is kept straight, the individual cannot get depressed. As simple as that. However, the problem is that putting this knowledge into practice is far from being simple. It requires a great deal of awareness. Just try it and you will know. As soon as your mind gets caught up in some thought process, your posture will stop being upright. The reaction is instantaneous and visible. As long as you are living in the moment, as long as you are aware, nothing can go wrong with your body. This awareness is really the true goal of yoga. But it takes dedicated and sincere practice. So use this book to start your own yoga practice. You will start working with the body, and ultimately find bliss. In *yogic* terms you will start from *vikshipta chitta* (diseased state of mind) and move towards *anandamaya chitta* (relaxed and blissful state of mind).

A few simple changes in the way you live your life will go a long way in relieving pain and strengthening your back. Let us start with when you wake up from the bed. Usually you wake up and immediately raise your back and jump straight out of bed, placing a tremendous load on the back. But observe how a cat wakes up. On waking, it first stretches out all the joints in the body, moves and stretches the back and then gingerly stands on its feet. Adopt a similar routine; stretch your body thoroughly, gently flex and twist your spine, move the joints and then roll onto one side and push yourself up. All of this will not take more than three minutes, but will help largely to keep you free from pulled and strained back muscles.

Practise a simple routine of yoga in the morning — a few stretches, few *asanas*, some *pranayama* and finally sit still for a few minutes listening to the birds chirping, watching the flowers or simply with your eyes closed. Yes, you can find time (half an hour, or even less) to do all of this. You will find your body complaining less, and that you are more relaxed and able to cope better with the demands of the day.

The *yogic* diet is a simple, light and fresh vegetarian meal. However it does not mean that you must turn vegetarian to practice yoga. Just try to eat light so that you feel light and full of life. If you are overweight then pay added attention to what you eat, and try to lose some weight, as we have seen, obesity is a major cause of backache.

Remember also that the condition of your back is closely related to your aging process. Having a supple, flexible back retards the aging process. Which is one of the fundamental reasons why people who practice yoga look so much younger.

Lastly, follow some basic codes of life. In yoga we call them *yama* and *niyama* — the basic rules by which to live a happy and peaceful life. They form the first two steps in the ladder of yoga. Some of them are *ahimsa* (non-violence), *aparigraha* (non-hoarding), *asteya* (non-stealing), *saucha* (cleanliness, internal and external) and so on. Following these simple principles will let you live a happy life, and keep you stress-free and relaxed, literally 'lifting a great burden off your back'.

5

Working on the Back

As we have seen, the back is an amazingly strong structure, which allows the spine to move in all directions and planes. The goal of this book is to first eliminate your backache and then to strengthen it so that your back remains pain-free, relaxed and supple. It's important not just to be free of your back pain, but also to have a strong and flexible back, which keeps you feeling light and healthy.

Do all the *asanas* mentioned in the following pages at your own pace and at your own level of flexibility. The goal is to slowly stretch the muscles in a way that they are not strained while doing something they may not have done in years. Start with the warm-up *asanas*. These will loosen all your joints and remove the basic stiffness in your spine and back. Then move to the strengthening *asanas*, which will improve the strength of the specific back muscles, the deep muscles of the back as well as the superficial muscles. Then move to the toning *asanas*, which improve the strength of the back as a whole. After completing this set, move to the stretching *asanas*, which remove knots and pains that might have occurred due to the heavy contractions that take place in the previous sets. Included in this set are a few *asanas* that use a bolster for assistance. These are extremely effective in removing aches and pains immediately. I have also included a set of partner stretches that will instantly remove pain from the back. This is particularly useful for people whose back is in pain right now and it is useful to have someone to assist them. Following this set, you can do the relaxation and meditation techniques which will calm you and rejuvenate you after the session.

Important point: Do remember that those who are in extreme pain should do the warm-up set and directly move to the stretching set, followed by partner stretches. Strengthening and toning should be gradually added to the programme only when the back is slowly becoming free of pain and strong enough so that it doesn't go into a spasm.

A) Warming Up

As mentioned before, it is crucial to warm up before the strenuous set of yogic exercises

TADASANA

- Stand with your feet 10 cms apart and your arms beside you. Raise your arms above your head and bring your palms together, stretch upwards and rise up on your toes. Balance your weight equally on both feet. Hold the position for 10 to 15 seconds. Inhale as you raise your arms and hold your breath as you hold the position and exhale as you come down. Repeat for five to 10 such rounds.

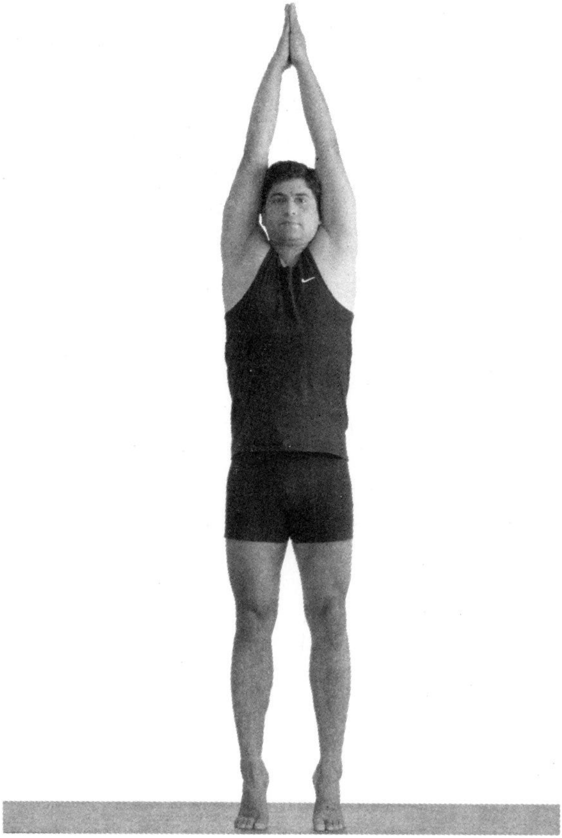

Tiryaka Tadasana

- Stand with your feet slightly apart. Lock your hands above your head and stretch upwards. Now exhale and bend sideways. Remember not to bend forward or backward but sideways and to keep your arms stretched out. Hold this position and your breath for a few seconds and then inhale and come up. Now repeat on the other side. Do five to 10 such rounds.

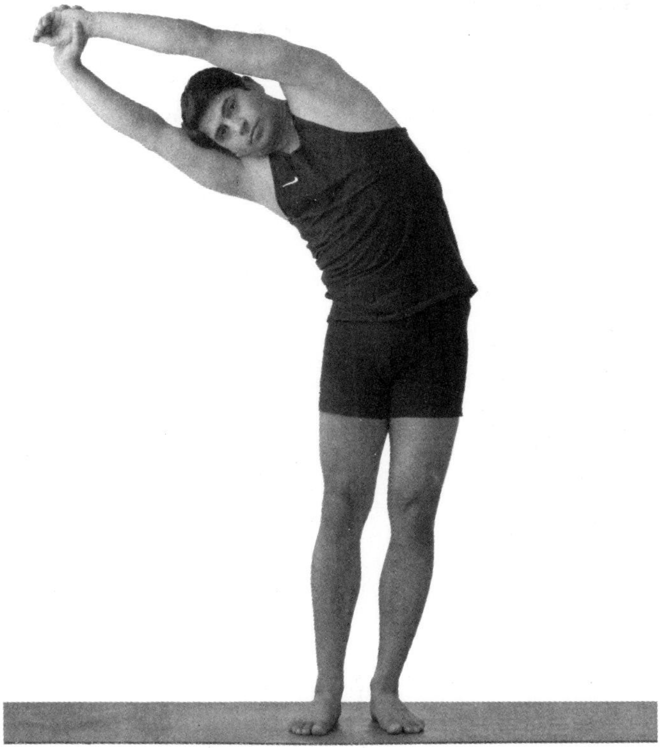

KATI CHAKRASANA

- Stand with your feet together and arms beside you. Wrap your left arm around your back and your right arm on your left shoulder. Now twist your body towards your left and push your left shoulder as far back as possible. Turn your head towards your left as well. Return to starting position and repeat the same on the other side. Repeat five to 10 such rounds. Exhale as you turn back; hold your breath as you hold the position and inhale as you come back.

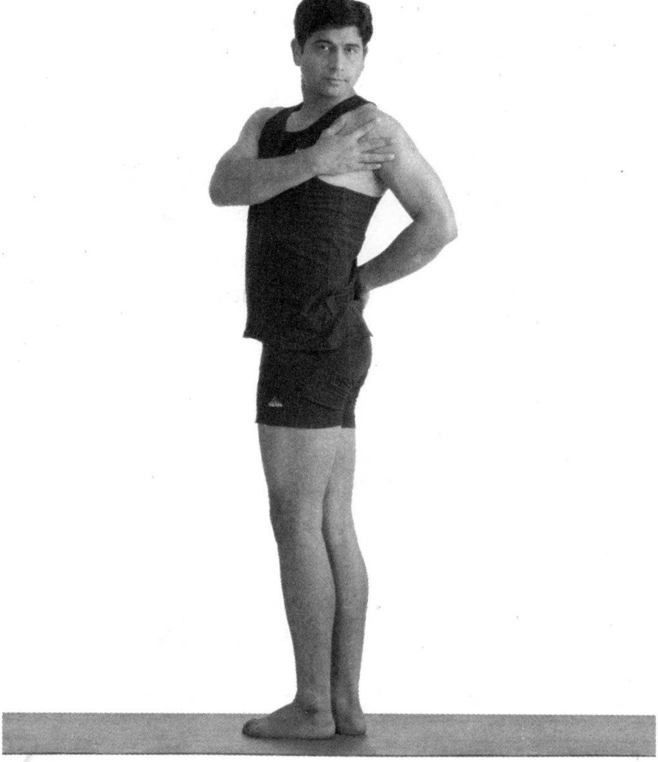

MARCHARIASANA

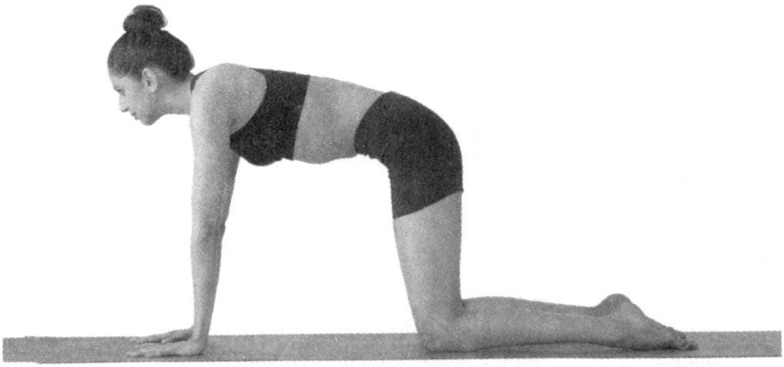

- Get down on all fours, keep your palms facing forward, directly under your shoulder and knees in line with your hips.

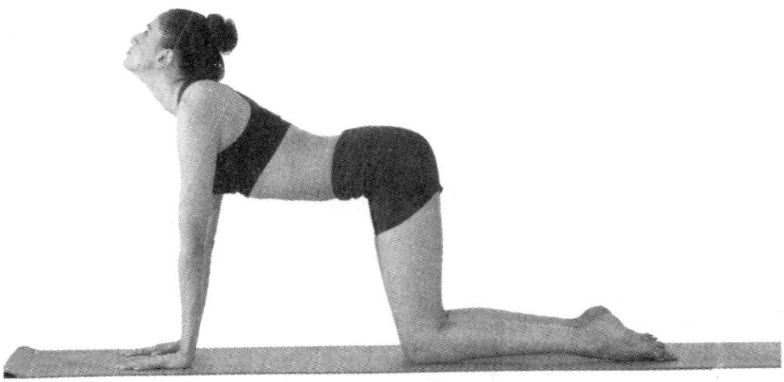

- Inhale and look up while you create an intense dip in your back. Hold the position and your breath for a few seconds.

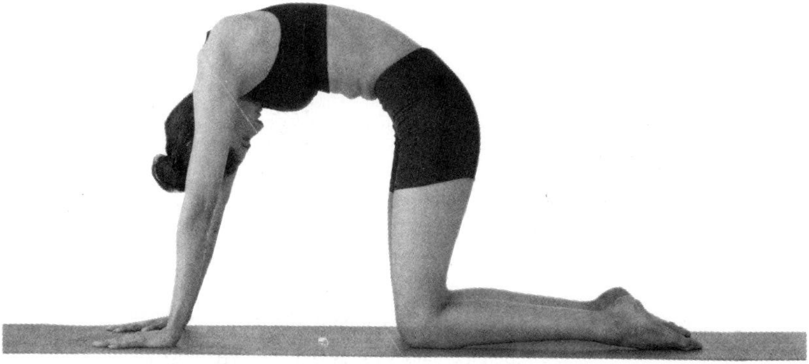

- Exhale and create an arch in your back. Hold your breath while you maintain the position for a few seconds. Do 10 to 15 rounds.

PASHIMOTTANASANA

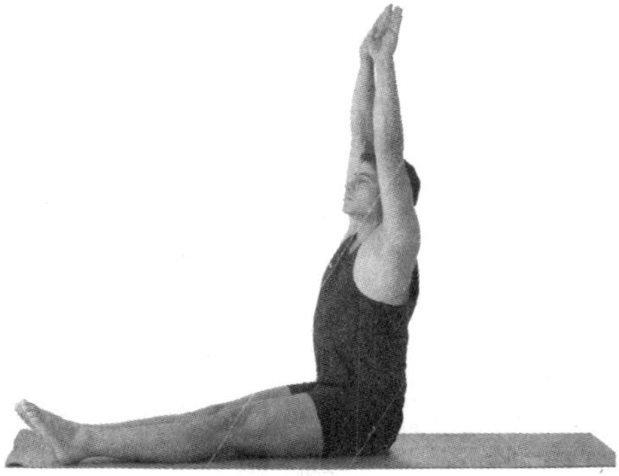

- Sit with your legs stretched out in front of you and your arms stretched above your head. Inhale as you raise your arms.

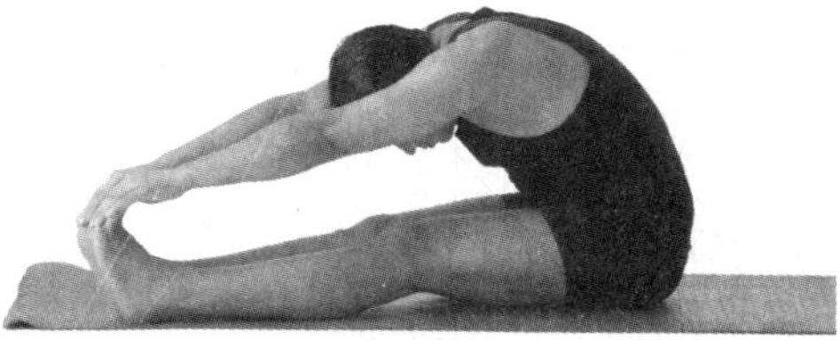

- Keeping your ears between your arms, bend forward to touch your toes. Exhale as you bend forward.

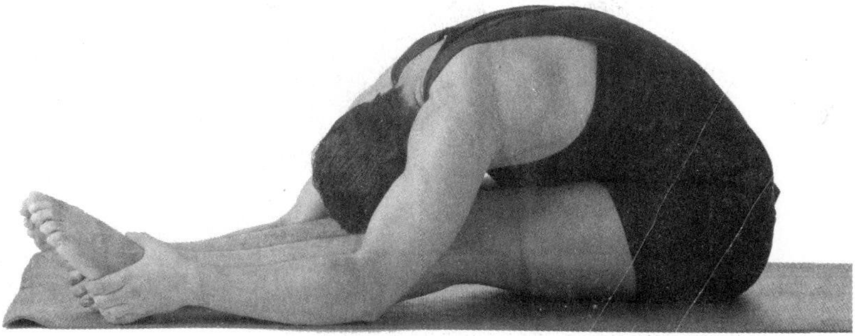

- Once you can comfortably touch your toes (over a period of time with daily practice), hold your ankle and place your forehead on your knees. Hold the position for a few seconds. Do 10 rounds.

B) Strengthening

Vipreet Naukasana Variation

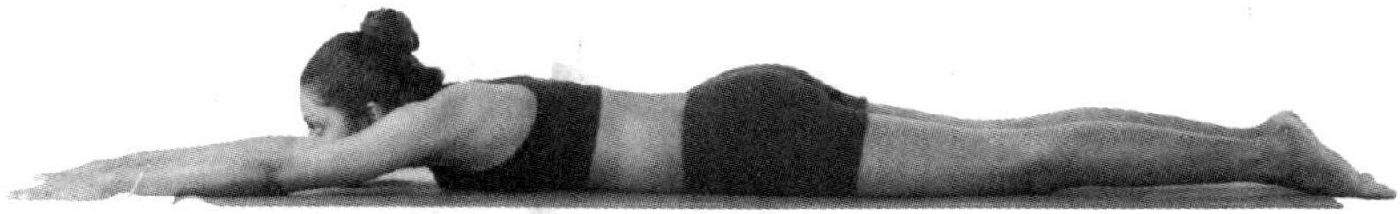

- Lie on your chest with your arms stretched in front of you and your legs stretched out, keeping your feet together.

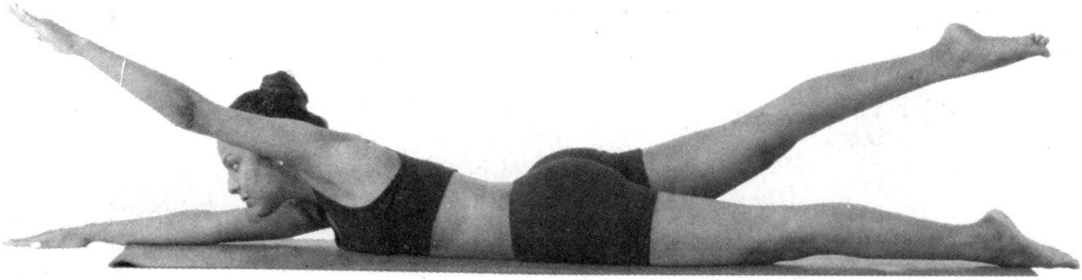

- Raise your left hand and your right leg up, keeping your hip on the ground. Keep your arm and leg straight. Hold for a few seconds, then bring them down and raise your right hand and left leg up. Repeat 10 to 15 rounds. Inhale as you raise your arms and exhale as you bring them down.

DHANURASANA

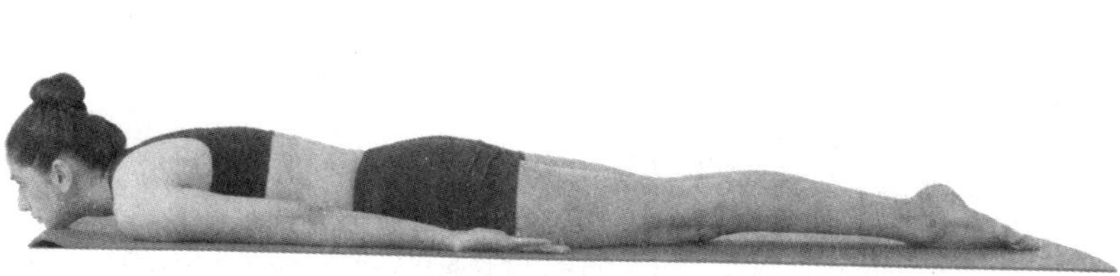

- Lie on you stomach with your hands beside you, chin on the floor and legs stretched straight.

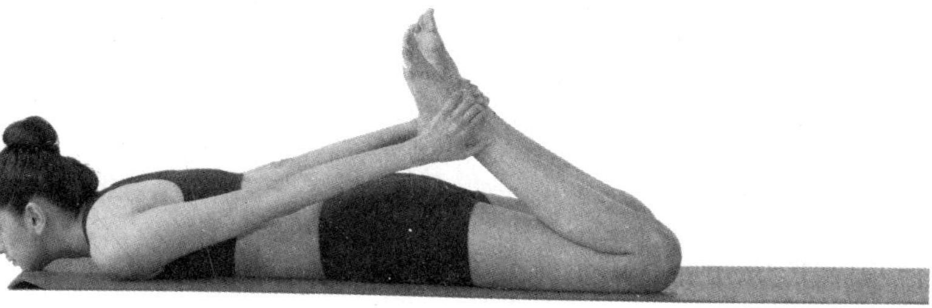

- Bend your knees and reach for you ankles and grip them firmly.

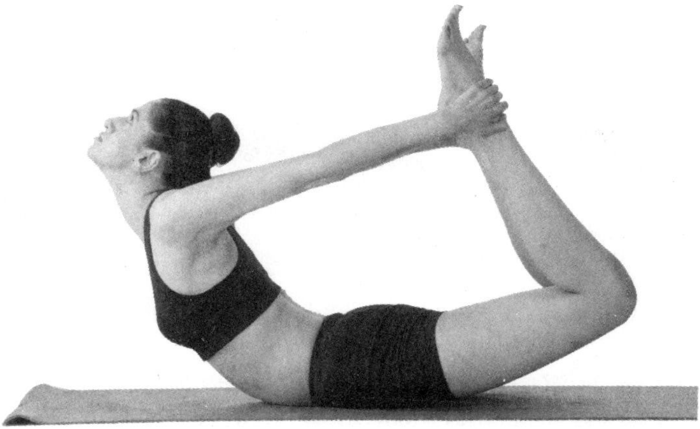

- Inhale and raise your upper body as high as possible by pushing your feet backwards. Hold the position for 10 to 20 seconds and then exhale and come down slowly.

Ek Pada Salabasana

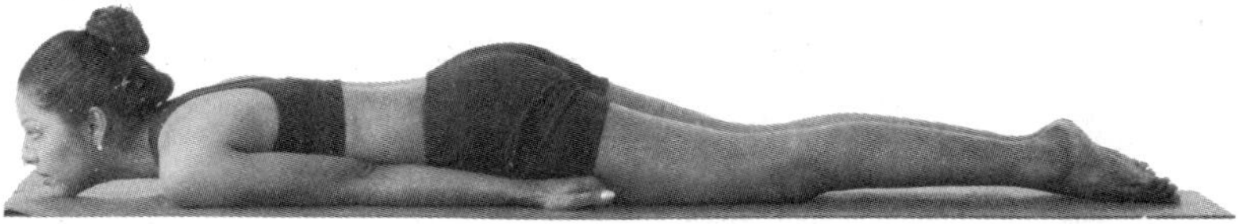

- Lie on your stomach with your chin on the floor. Make your palms into fists and place them palms facing down under your thigh.

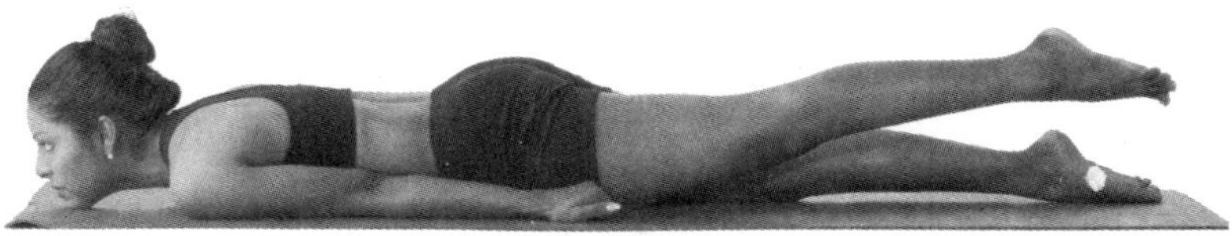

- Inhale and raise one leg up. Keep your awareness on your lower back.

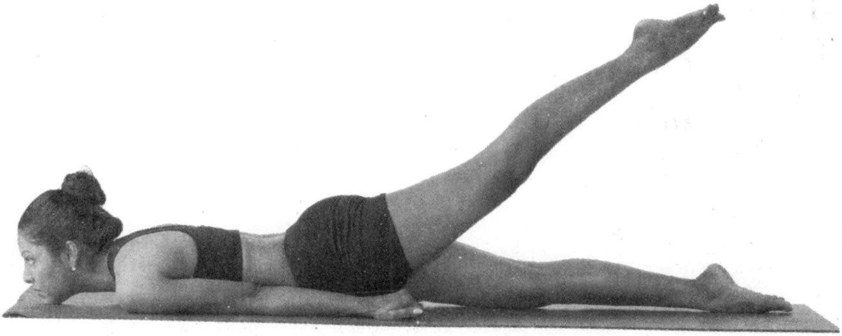

- Raise your leg up as high as possible and hold the position for a few seconds. Exhale and bring the leg down and do the same with the other leg. Do five to 10 rounds.

Dwi Pada Salabasana

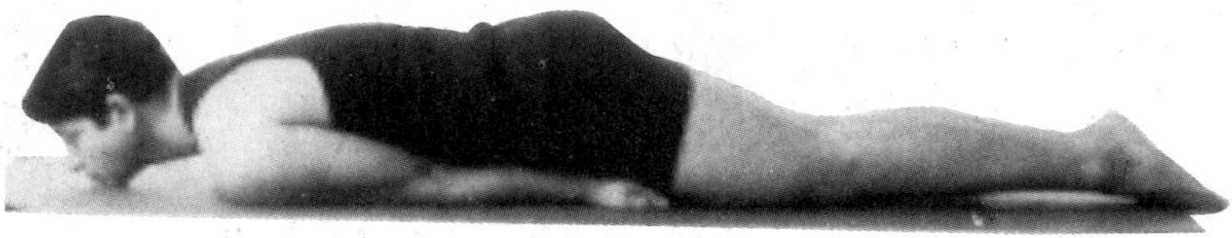

- Lie on your stomach with your chin on the floor. Make your palms into fists and place them palm facing down under your thigh.

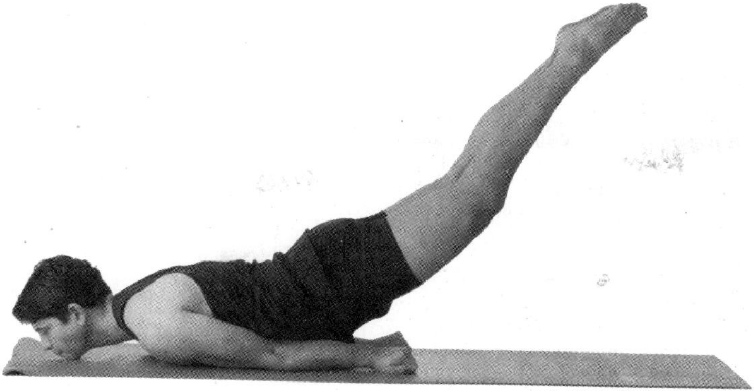

- Inhale and raise both your legs off the floor as high as possible. Hold the position for a few seconds, then exhale and come down slowly.

BHUJANGASANA

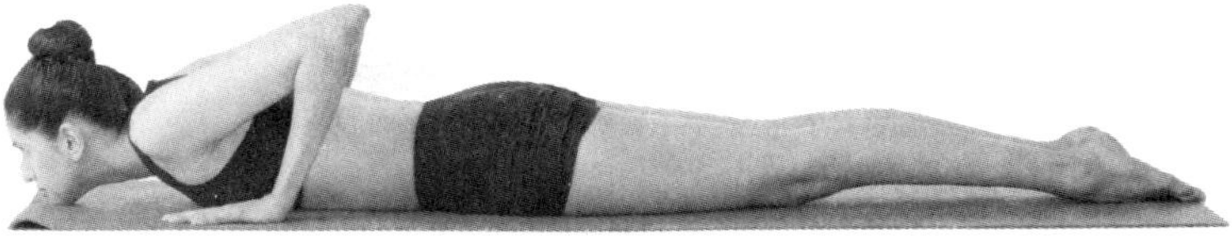

- Lie on your stomach with your hands beside you at chest level and feet together.

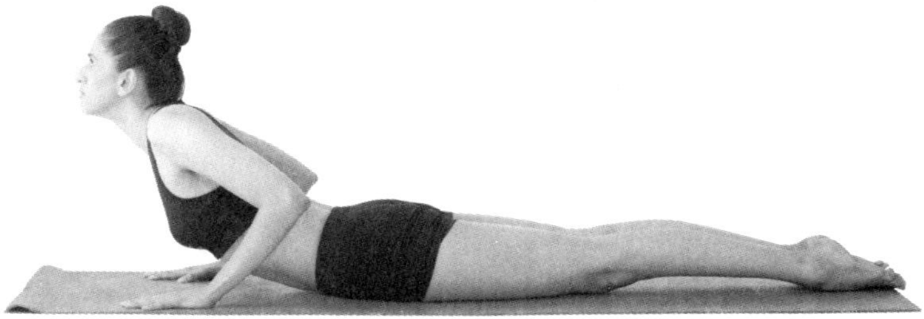

- Inhale and raise your upper body up slightly. Hold the position for a few seconds.

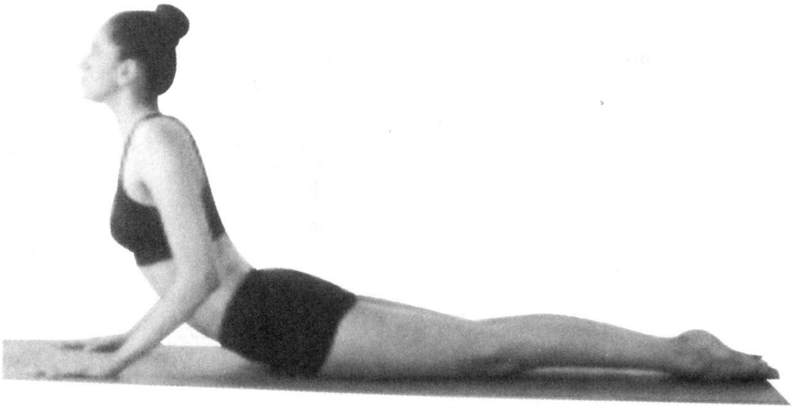

- Raise your body up as much as possible and hold the position for 10 to 15 seconds. Keep your shoulders back and hold your breath. Exhale and lower your body.

VARIATION 1

- Lie on your stomach as in *bhujangasana* to start. Now raise your upper body and your palms off the floor. Stretch your arms behind your back as far as possible and hold the position for 10 to 15 seconds. Remember to keep your feet together. Hold your breath as you raise your body. Remain static while you hold the position and exhale before lowering your body.

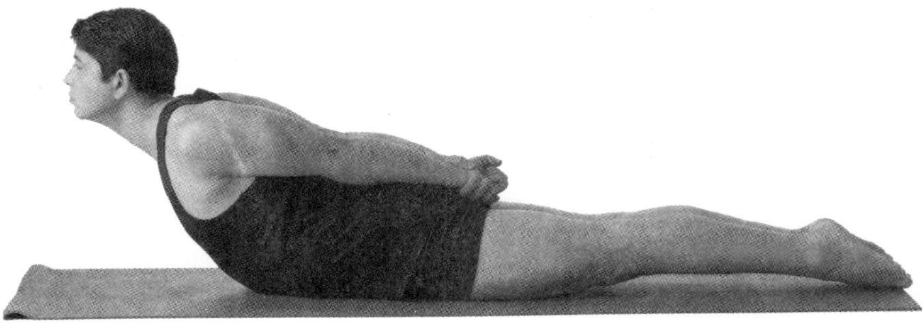

Variation 2

- Lie on your stomach with legs together and hands beside your chest. Bend your knees and bring your feet towards your bottom. Come up on your elbows and support your chin on your palms. Take your focus to your back and hold position for a few seconds. Inhale as you raise your torso and exhale as you come down.

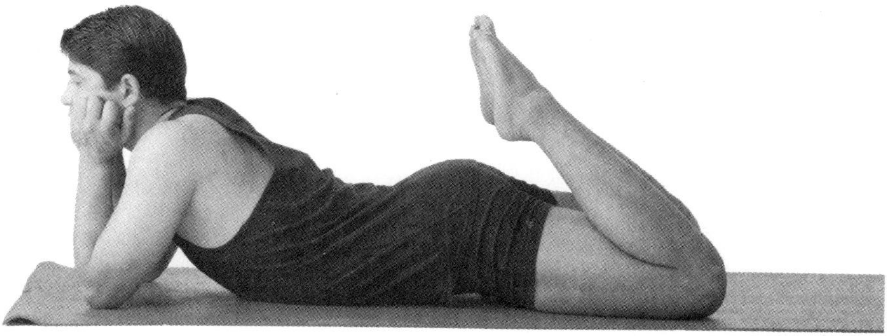

VARIATION 3

- Lie in the starting position as in *bhujangasana,* keeping your palms on the ground at chest level. Bend your knees and then raise your upper body so that your elbows are straight. Drop your head back. Hold the position and your breath for a few seconds; exhale and lower your torso and then your legs.

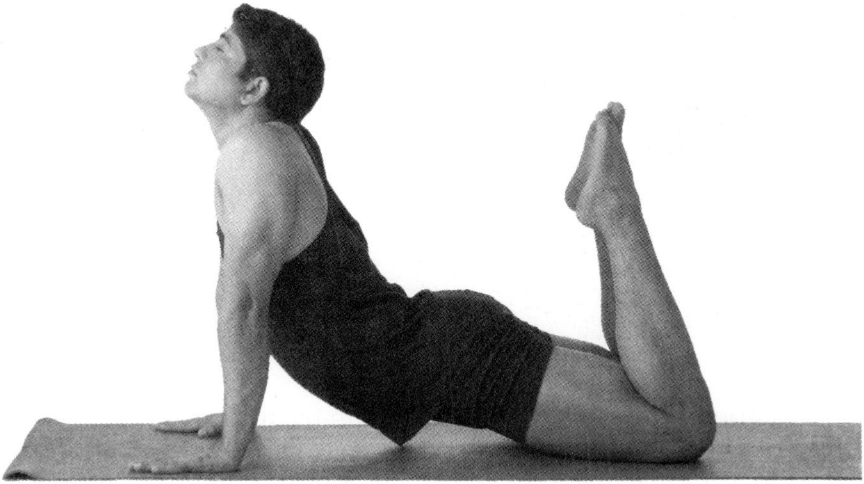

VARIATION 4

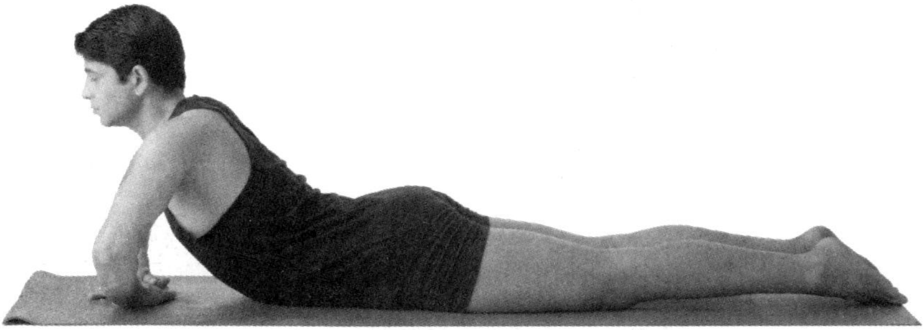

- Interlock your palms and place them facing downward on the ground at chest level. Support yourself well on your arms. Keep your feet together.

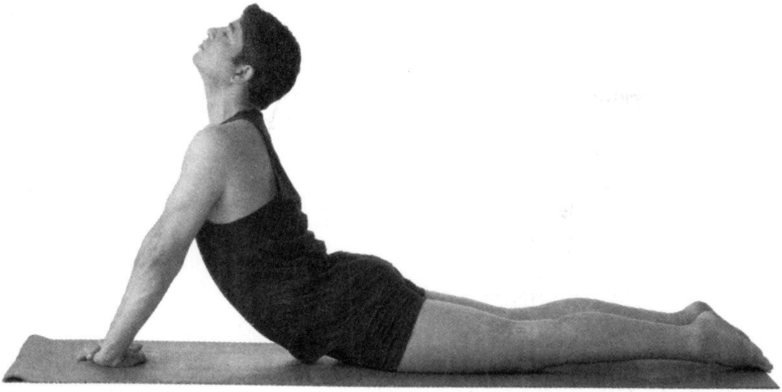

- Inhale and straighten your elbows so that you get a contraction in your back and a stretch in your abdomen. Drop your head back and hold the position and your breath for a few seconds. Exhale and lower your body.

Triyaka Bhujangasana

- Lie on your stomach with hands beside you at chest level. Inhale, raise your upper body and straighten your elbows. Now twist your torso to the left and attempt to look back at your feet. Hold this position for a few seconds and then come back to the centre and lower your torso to the ground. Repeat the same on your right side. Hold your breath while you maintain the position and exhale as you lower your body.

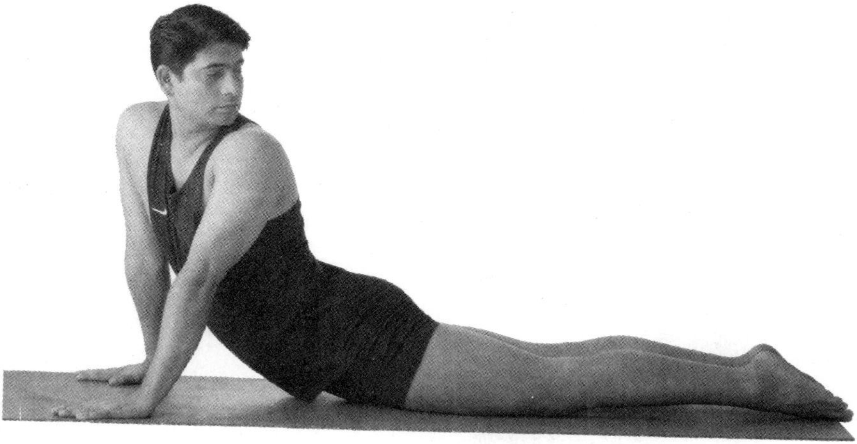

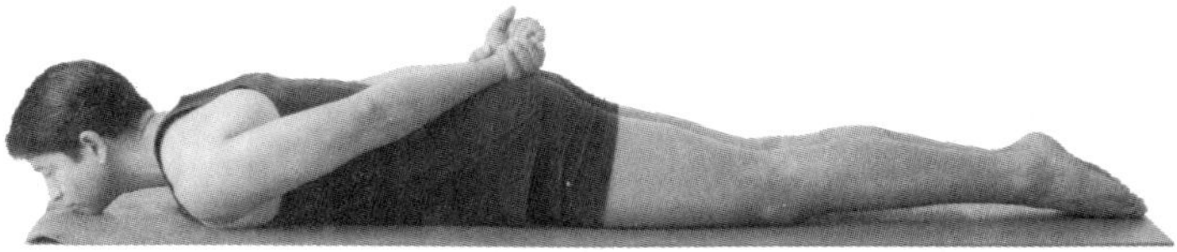

- Lie on your stomach with your chin on the floor, feet together and your hands locked behind your back.

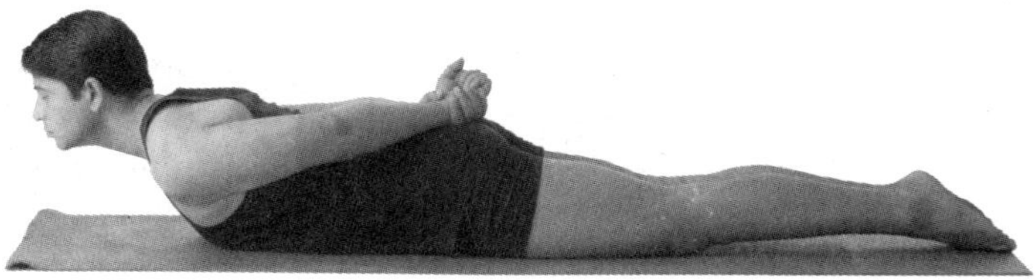

- Inhale and raise your upper body, keeping the hands locked.

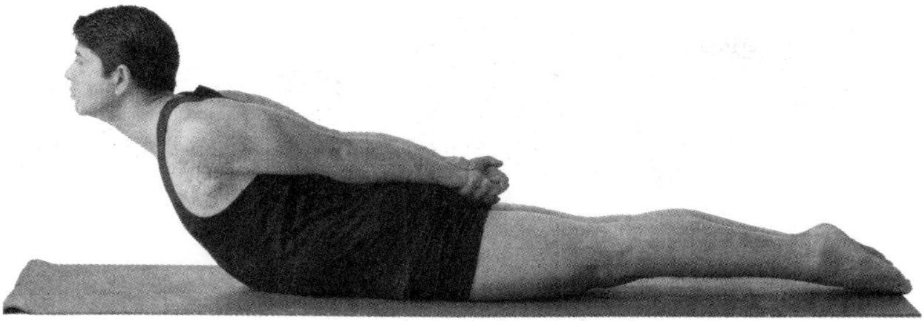

- Pull your arms as far back as possible towards your bottom, raising your upper body higher and dropping your head back. Hold the position for a few seconds. Hold your breath as you maintain the position and exhale and come down.

MERUDANDASANA (PRONE LINE)

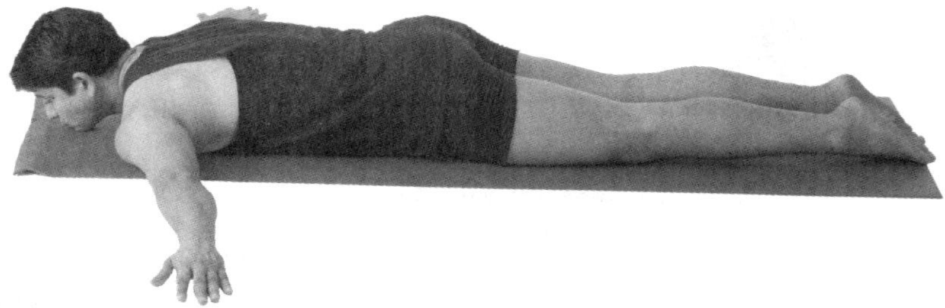

- Lie on your stomach with your hands at shoulder level and feet together.

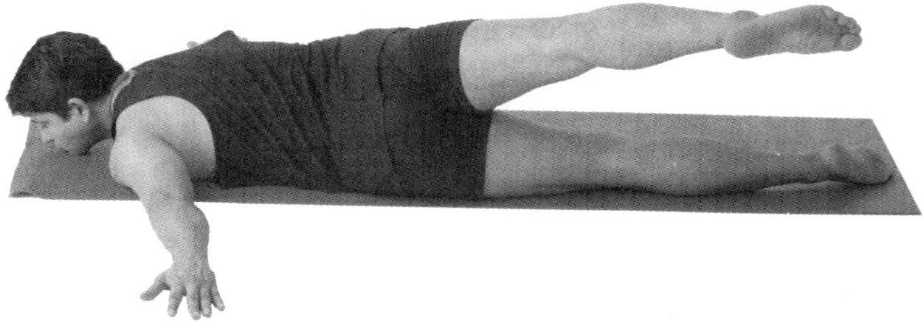

- Inhale and lift your right leg. Keep your shoulders on the floor as far as possible.

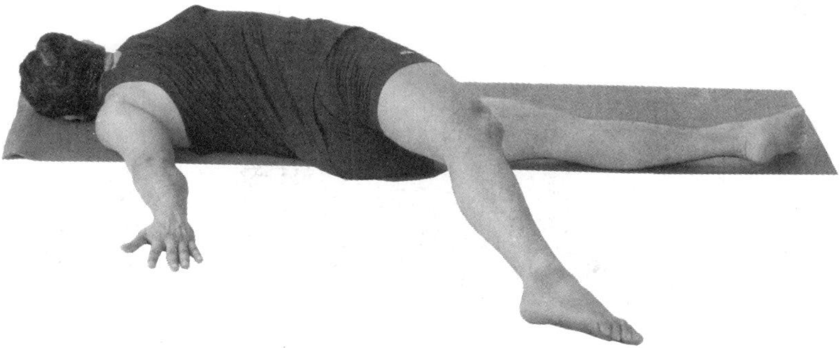

- Place the right leg on the floor across the left leg. Turn your face towards the right and keep the left leg straight. Remember to keep both the shoulders on the floor. Hold the position for a few seconds and then change the leg and repeat.

SETUBANDHASANA

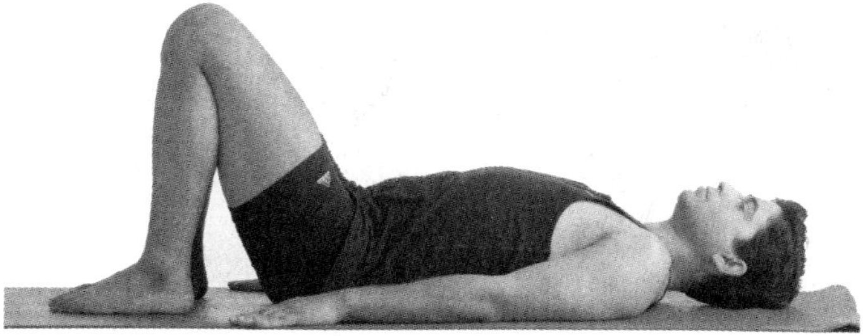

- Lie on your back with your knees up and your hands placed beside you. Your feet are placed perpendicular to the floor.

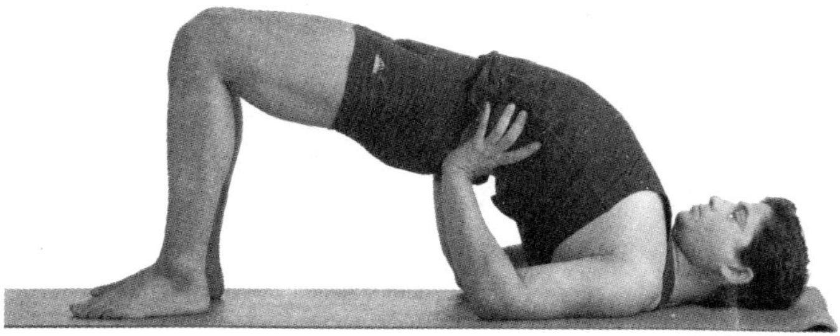

- Lift your bottom and support it with your hands. Bring your awareness to the arch created in your back and hold the position for a few seconds and then lower your bottom. If you are comfortable in this position, then you may move to the following stage.

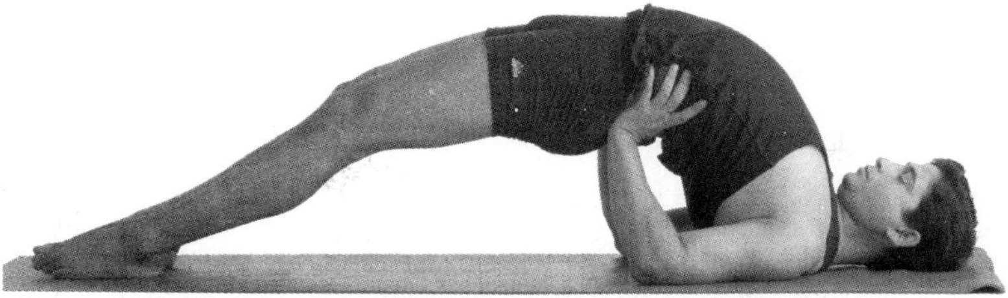

- Support yourself well on both your hands, then gently begin to walk your feet forward till they are straight. Hold position for a few seconds, then walk your feet back to the second stage. Lift your bottom off your hands and lower it.

C) Toning

Place both hands behind the head and raise.

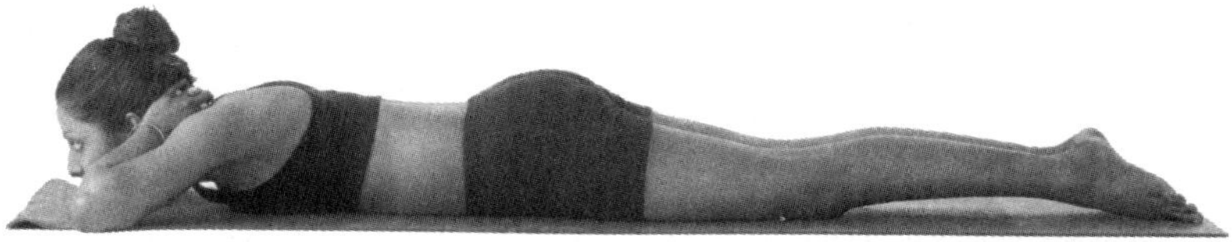

- Lie on your stomach with your hands interlocked behind your neck and your legs straight.

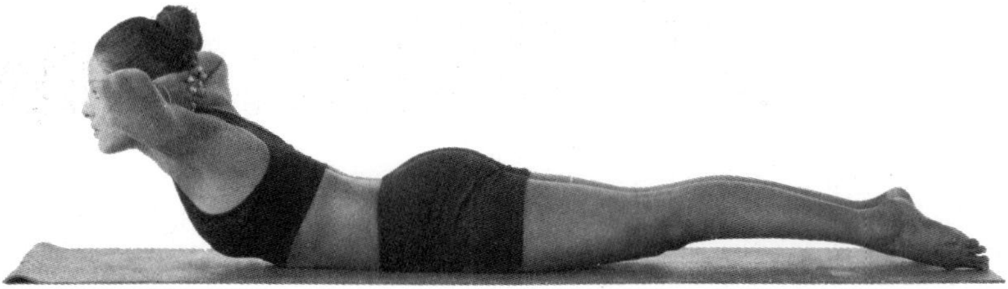

- Inhale and raise your upper body as high as you can comfortably do so. Exhale and lower your body to the ground. Do 10 to 15 rounds.

Viprit Naukasana

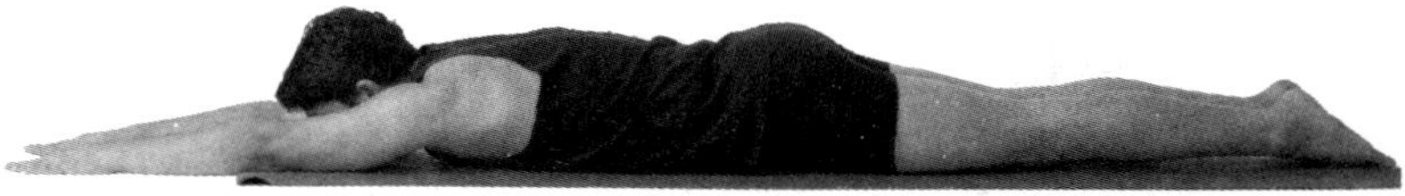

- Lie on your stomach with the legs together and arms stretched out above your head.

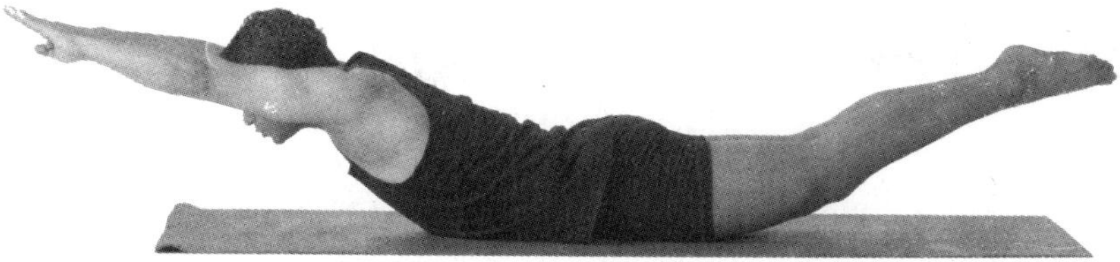

- Inhale and lift your arms and your legs up as high as possible and hold the position for a few seconds and then lower them. Repeat to do five or six rounds.

D) Stretching

Merudandasana-Variation 1

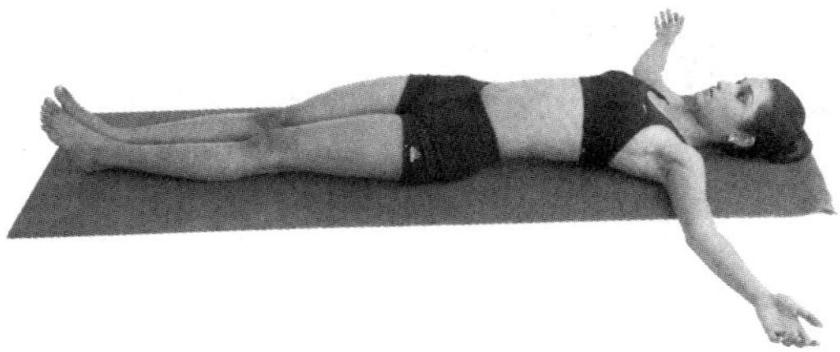

- Lie flat on your back with arms at shoulder level.

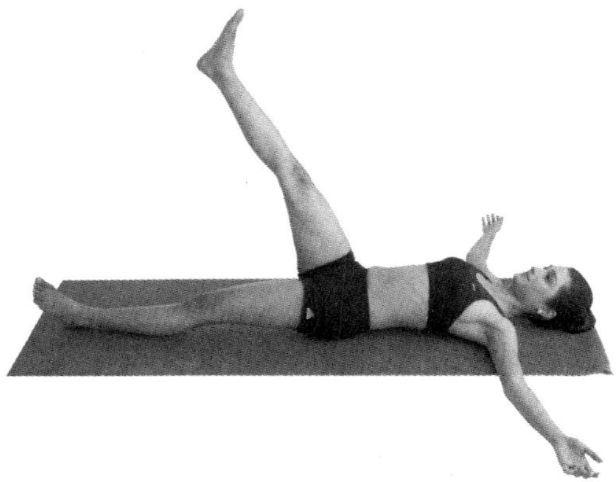

- Raise one leg up.

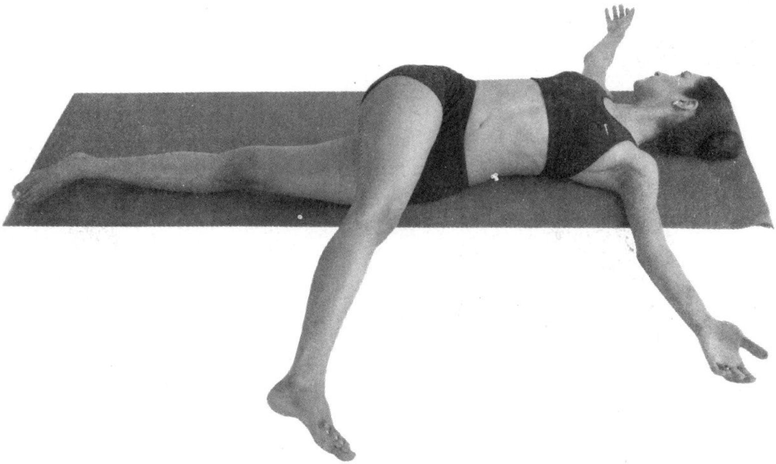

- Place the leg on the opposite side keeping your knees straight. Remember to keep both shoulder's on the floor and look in the opposite direction. Bring your awareness to relaxing your back. Return to starting position and change the leg. Breathe normally.

VARIATION 2

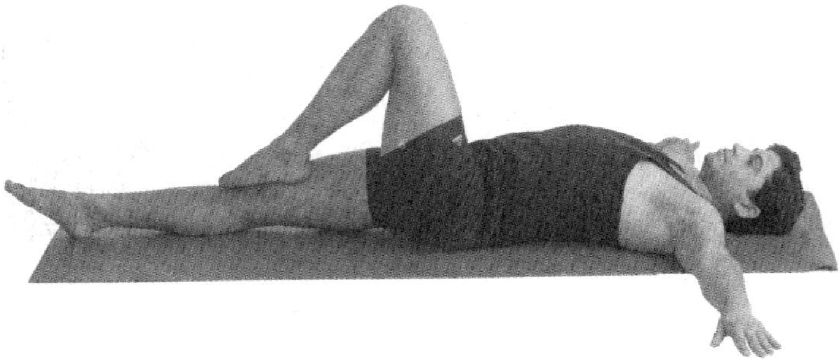

- In starting position, lie flat on your back with arms outstretched at shoulder level. Place one foot on the other knee.

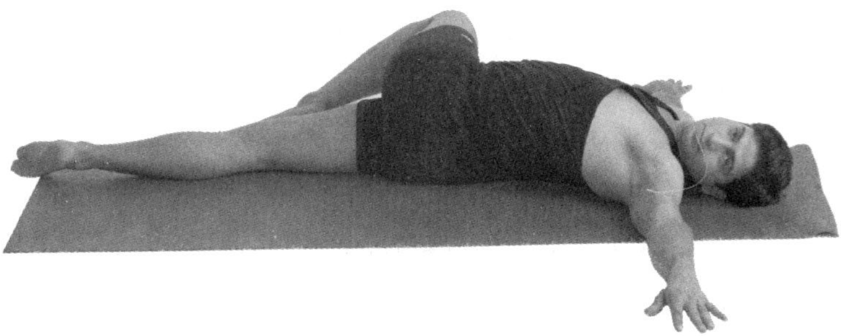

- Drop the upright knee to the opposite side. Keep both shoulders on the floor. Look in the opposite direction.

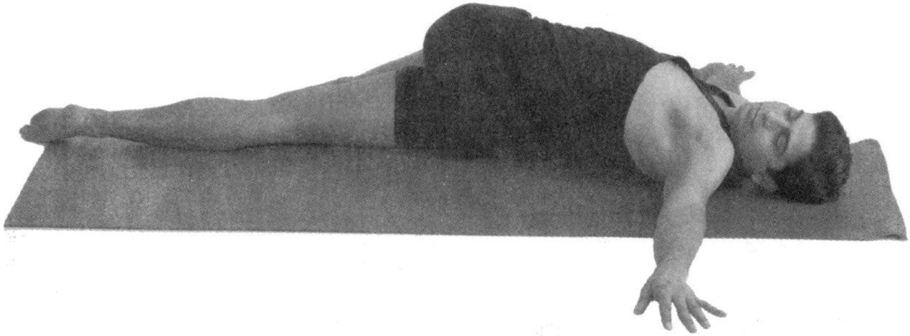

- Try to place the knee on the floor. Focus on keeping the shoulder down. Hold the position for a few seconds. Return to starting position and do the same on the opposite side. Breathe normally while holding the stretch.

PAVANMUKTASANA

Lie flat on your back with your hands beside you.

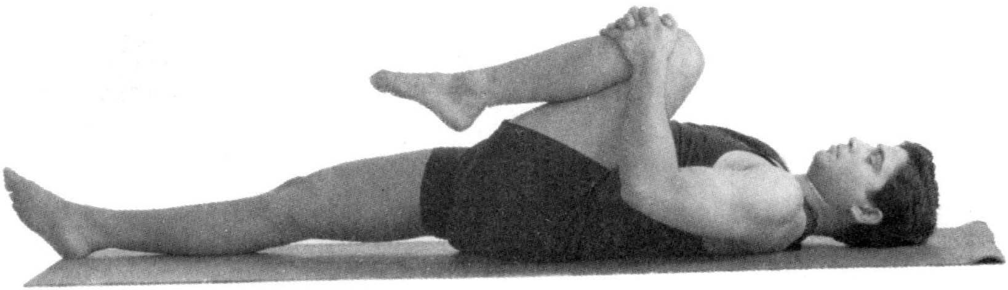

- Bring your one knee up and hold it with both hands. Hug it close to your chest and hold the position while focusing on relaxing your lower back.

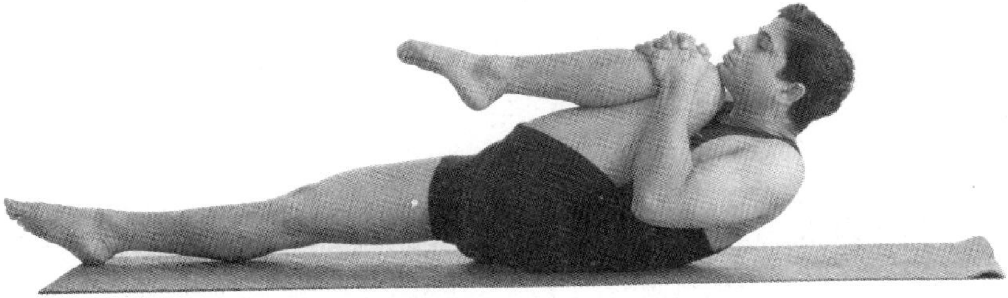

- Raise your chin up to touch your knee. Hold the position for a few seconds, then return to the starting position and repeat the same with the other leg. Breathe normally while you hold the position.

Dwipada Pawanmuktasana

Lie on your back with hands beside you.

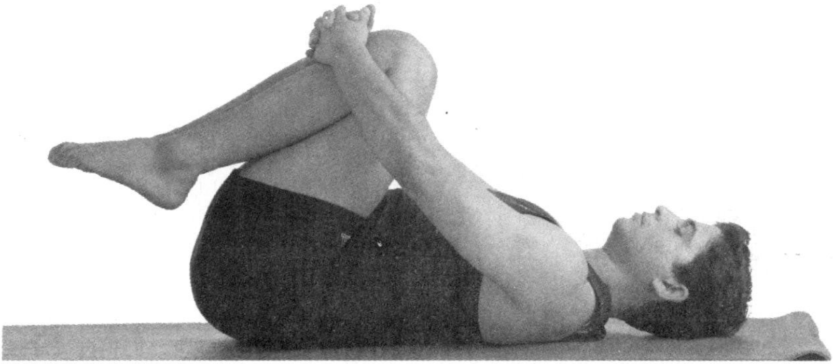

- Draw both your knees up towards your chest.

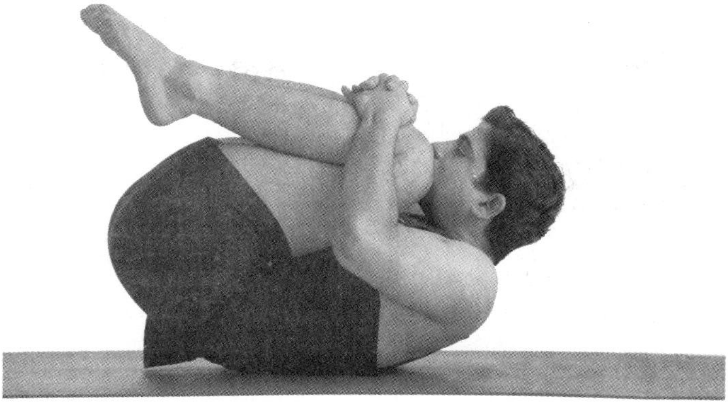

- Draw them up as close as possible to your chest and then bring your chin to meet your knees. Hold the position for a few seconds. Breathe normally while you hold this position. Then rock back and forth a few times in the same position to massage your lower back.

PADAMASANA (WITH HANDS BEHIND AND STRETCH)

- Sit in *padmasana* or simply with your legs crossed. Place one palm over the other and hold one wrist. Drop your head back and straighten and lift your arms up enough to feel a contraction in your upper back. Hold the position for a few seconds. Repeat five to six times.

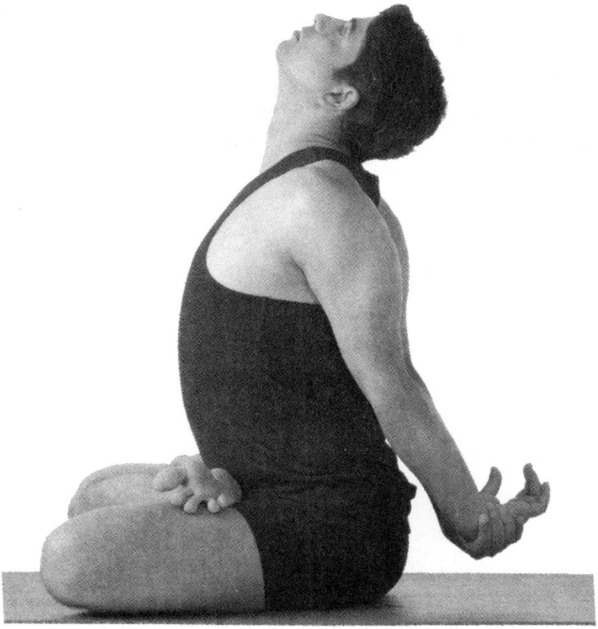

Bolster Stretch 1

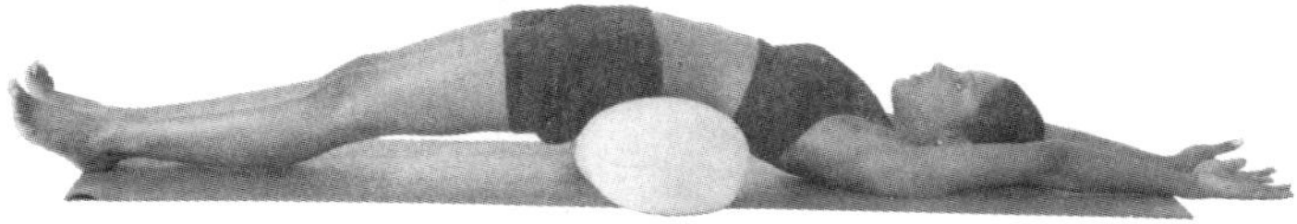

- Place the bolster on the floor and lie on it with your lower back resting directly on the bolster. Stretch your hands above your head and straighten your legs and relax in this position for a while.

Bolster Stretch 2

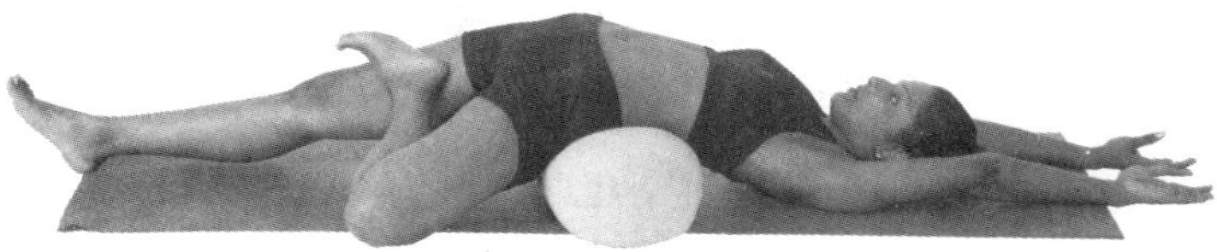

- Sit with the bolster behind you. Place your left ankle on your right thigh and gently lower yourself on to the bolster. The arc of your lower back should rest on the bolster. Relax in this position for a while and then repeat the same with the right ankle on the left thigh.

Bolster Stretch 3

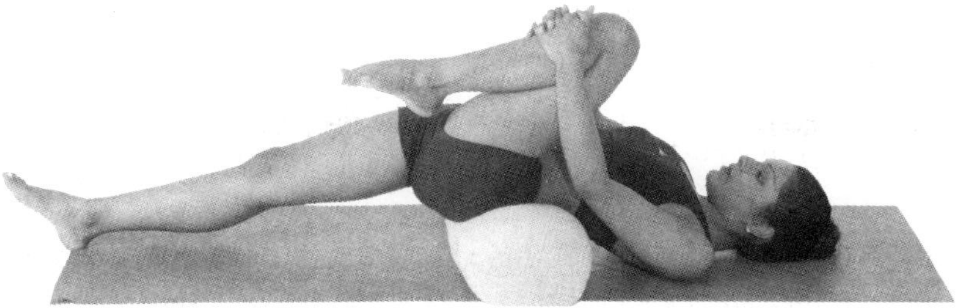

- Lie on the bolster with your lower back resting on it. Draw up your left knee to your chest and hold the position for a few seconds. Repeat the same with your right knee.

E) Partner Stretching

Stretch 1

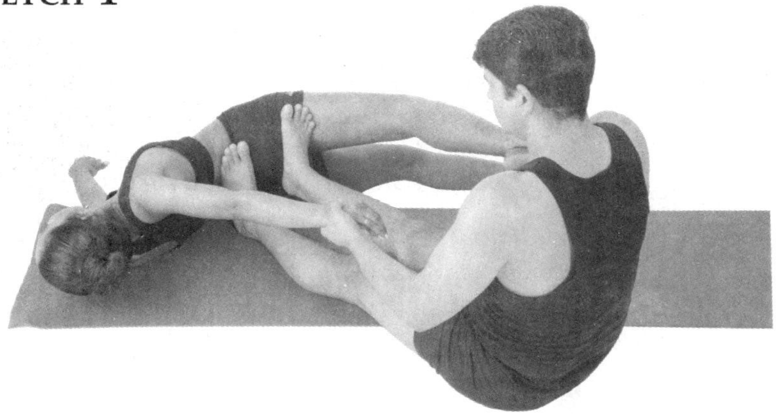

- Make the partner lie on her side. Hold the top arm and leg. Massage her sides, lower back and gluteus with your foot. Gently walk up and down her sides. Check with your partner and see that you put the right amount of pressure so as to relax the muscles.

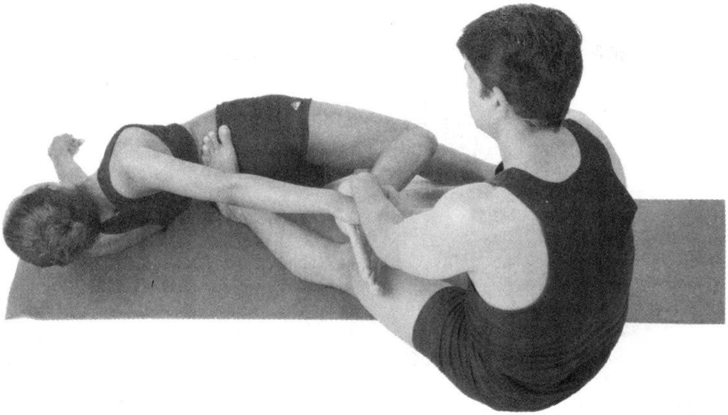

- Make your partner hold her ankle and then you hold her ankle and put your foot on her back and push forward so as to give her a good stretch in the back. Begin gently and increase pressure gradually, making sure to check your partner's comfort. Now do the same on the other side of her body.

STRETCH 2

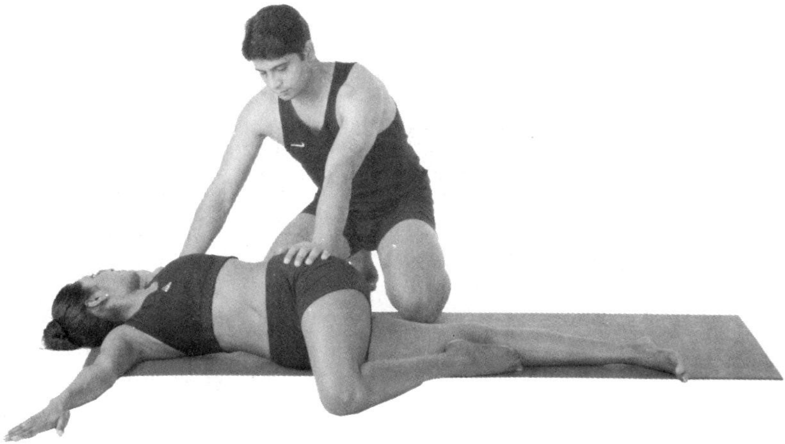

- Make your partner lie on her back, flat with arms stretched at shoulder level. Place one foot on one knee and gently drop the other knee to the opposite side while all the while keeping the shoulders on the floor. Now put your hand just below the waist and push towards the knee that's on the ground. Your partner should get a twist in her back. Check with your partner on how far you can push. Hold the stretch for a count of 10.

STRETCH 3

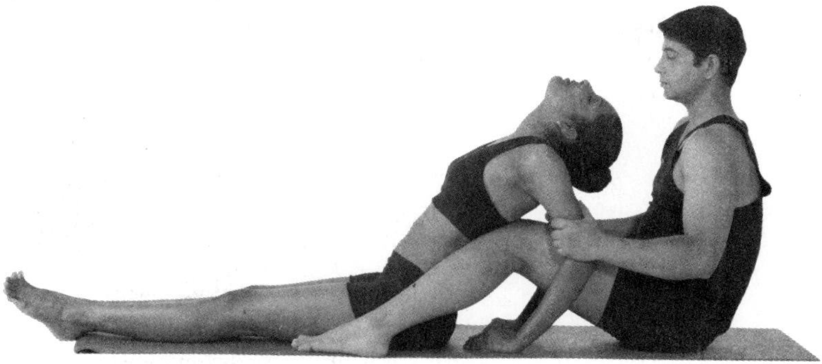

- Make your partner sit between your legs with her legs outstretched. Place your knees on either side of the spine and ask your partner to fall back towards you. Hold her arms and pull as far back as is comfortable for her. Hold the stretch for a count of 10.

STRETCH 4

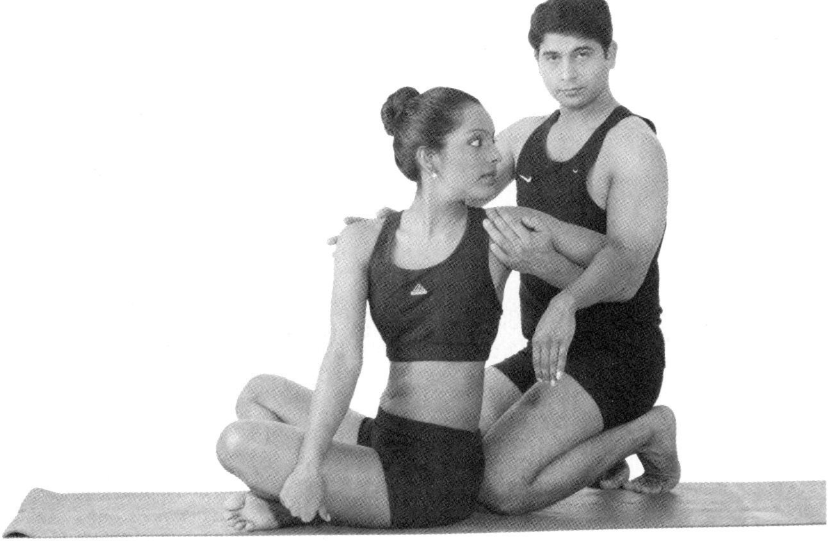

- Make your partner sit cross-legged and you sit on her side. Now hold the shoulder that is away from you with one hand and pull it towards you while you hold the other shoulder and push it away from you. This will twist the torso and relax the back. Check with your partner about how far you can twist. Hold the stretch for a count of 10.

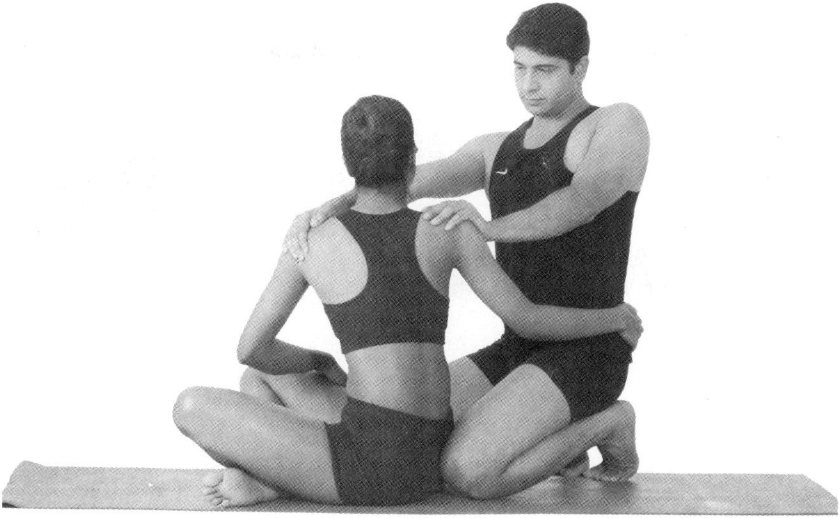

- Turn you partner the other way and do the same. Place your partner's arms across your waist, push the shoulder that you pulled earlier and vice versa, giving an equal twist on the opposite side. Hold the stretch to a count of 10.

STRETCH 5

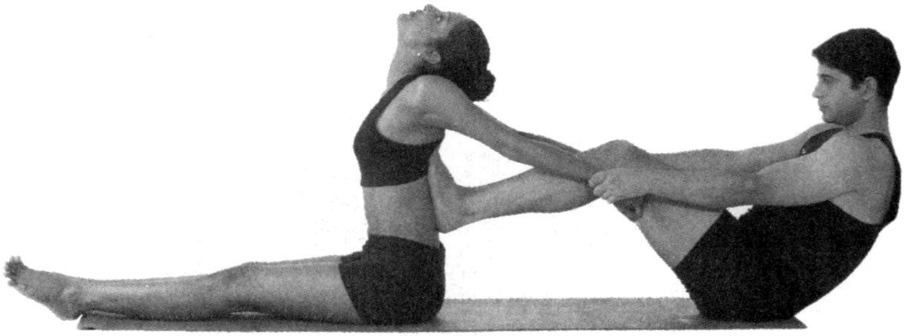

- Make your partner sit in front of you with the legs outstretched. Sit behind her and hold her wrists. Place your feet on either side of the spine in the middle back and gently begin to straighten your legs, pushing them forward. Ask your partner to drop her head back and relax. Hold the stretch for a count of 10.

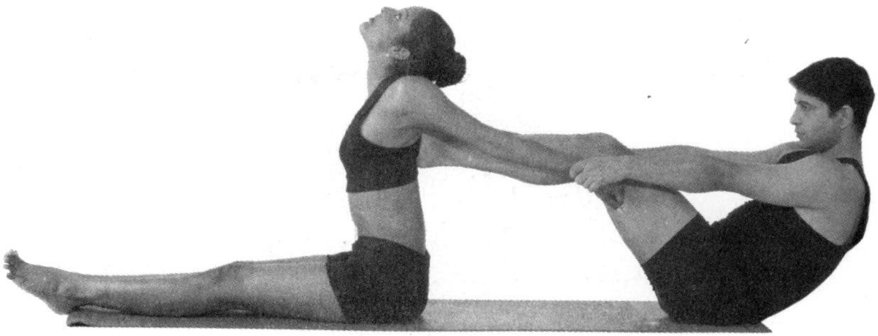

- Place your feet on either side of the spine of the upper back and gently straighten your legs. Ask your partner to relax and drop her head back. Hold the stretch for a count of 10.

STRETCH 6

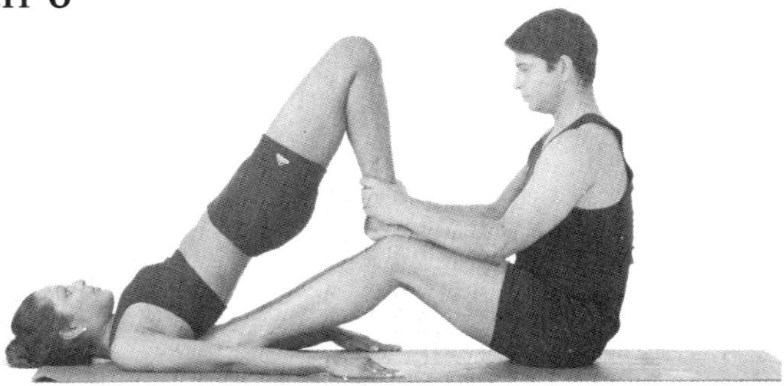

- Make your partner lie on her back with hands beside her. Place her feet on your knees and ask her to lift her bottom off the floor, while you slide your legs under her shoulders.

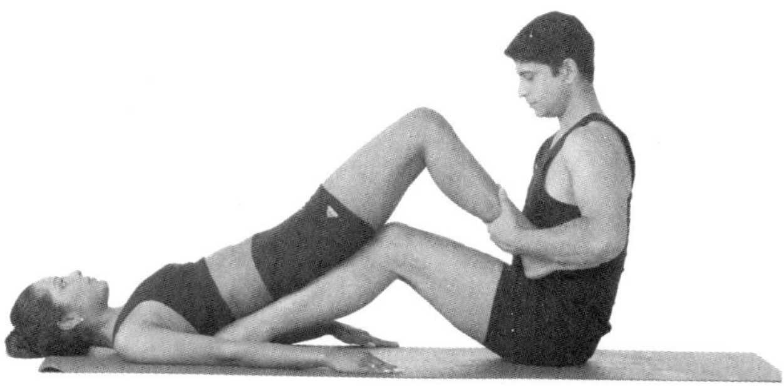

- Rest her back and bottom on your legs and pull them forward slightly.

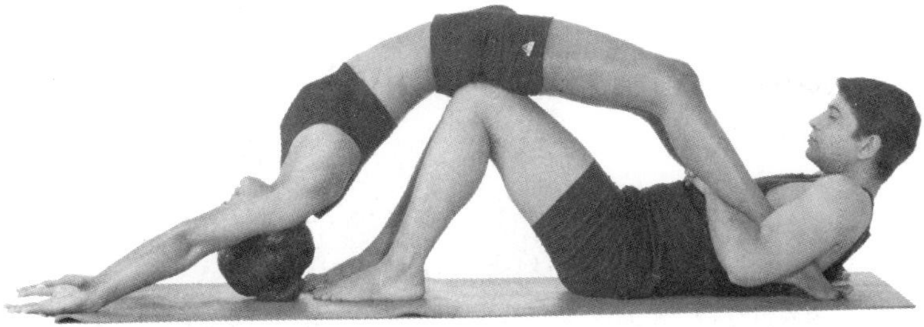

- Rest the top of the bottom on your knees and raise your knees higher so that you lift them off the floor. Hold her feet firmly as you fall back to give them a stretch in the back. Ask your partner to relax and allow her body to hang loose. Hold the stretch for a count of 10.

Stretch 7

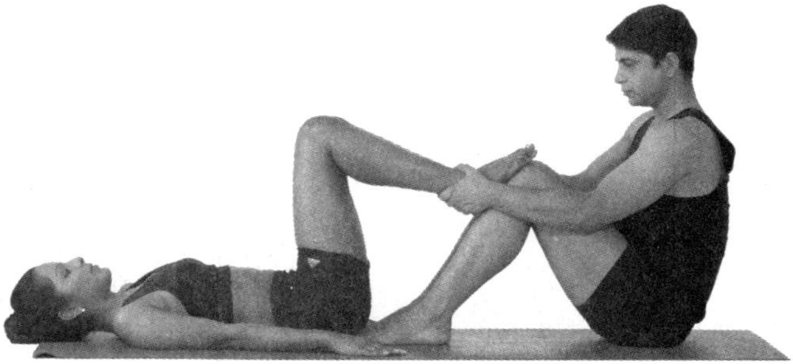

- Ask your partner to lie on her back and place her feet on your knees.

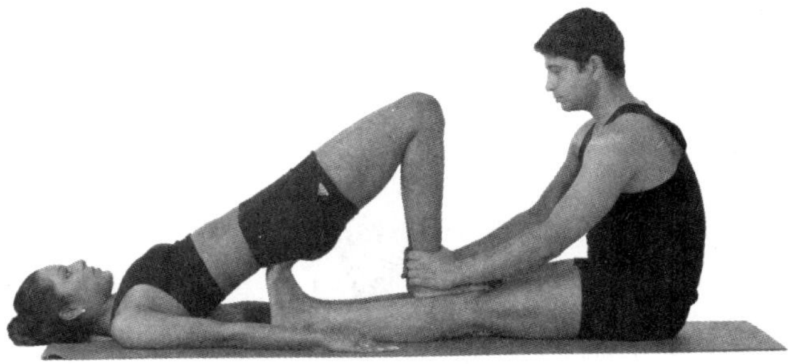

- Straighten your knees and ask your partner to lift her bottom off the floor as you slide your feet and place them on the lower back. Remember to rest her back on the balls of your toes and not directly on the toes as it could be uncomfortable.

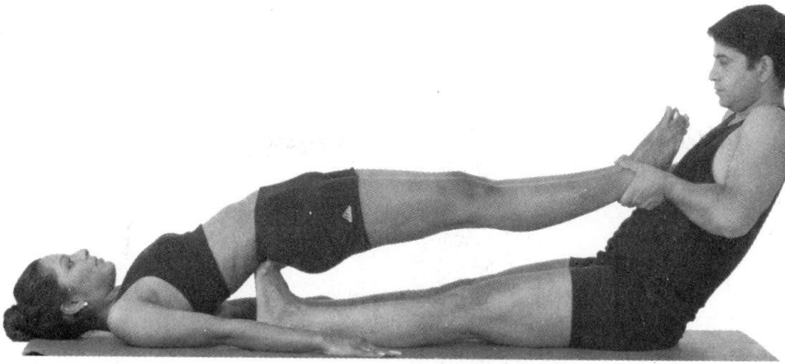

- Hold her feet and pull her towards yourself, stretching the lower back.

STRETCH 8

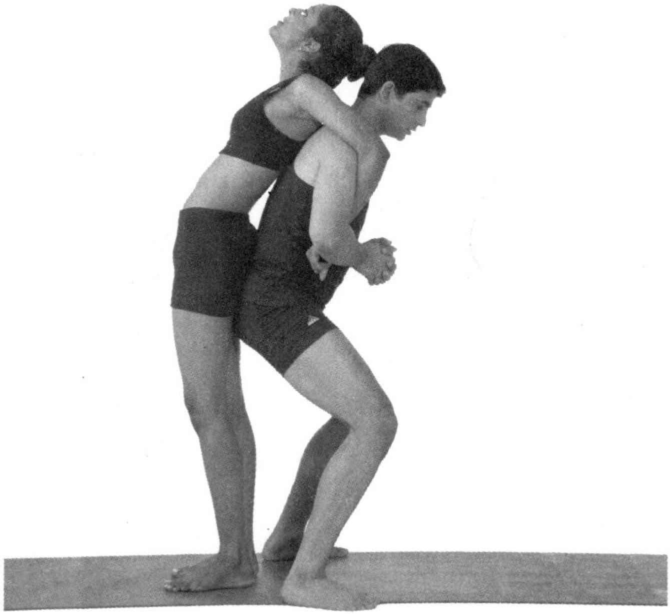

- Stand back to back with your partner. Lock her hands with yours over your shoulders and place your bottom just below your partner's. You might have to bend your knees to accommodate this.

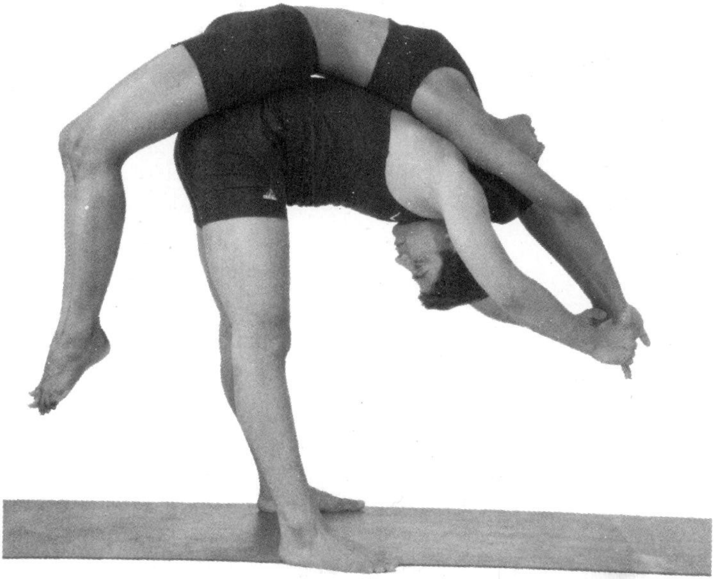

- Bend you back and lift your partner off the floor. Stretch her hands over your head and rock her gently from head to toe. Bend your knees and bring her down gently. Ask her to bend forward and touch her toes for a few seconds.

Simple Back Massage

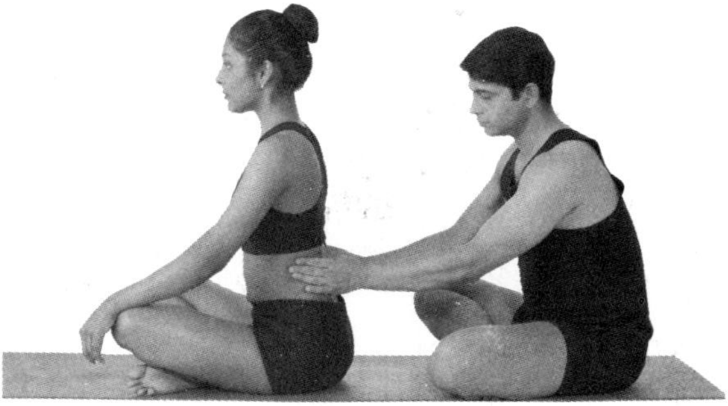

- Massage your partner's back, starting with the shoulders. Use your palm and your fingers to gently knead the muscles.

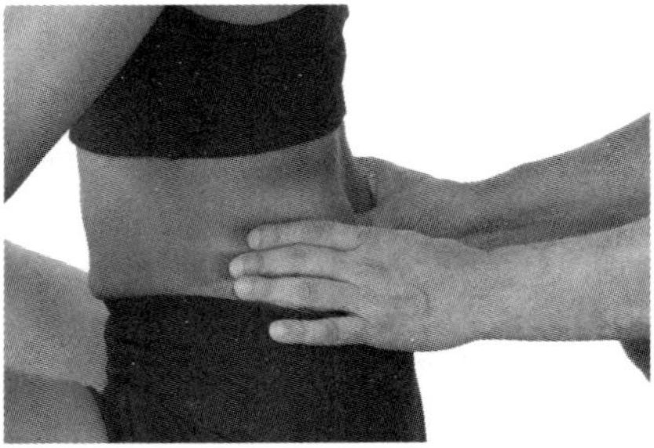

- Use your fingers and gently massage the muscles on either side of the spine and all along the spine.

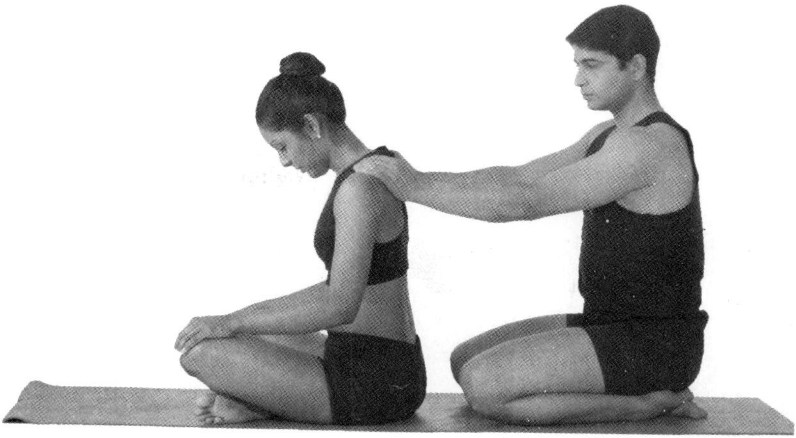

- Pay close attention to the lower back while massaging the same way.

F) Relaxation and Meditation

Cool down the body with these simple set of yogic *asanas*.

Sahaj Pranayama

- Sit in *vajrasana* and close your eyes, keeping your back straight and your hands on your knees. Take in a deep breath, hold and press your chin to the neck. Hold your breath for five seconds and come up and exhale through the mouth. Repeat 15 times.

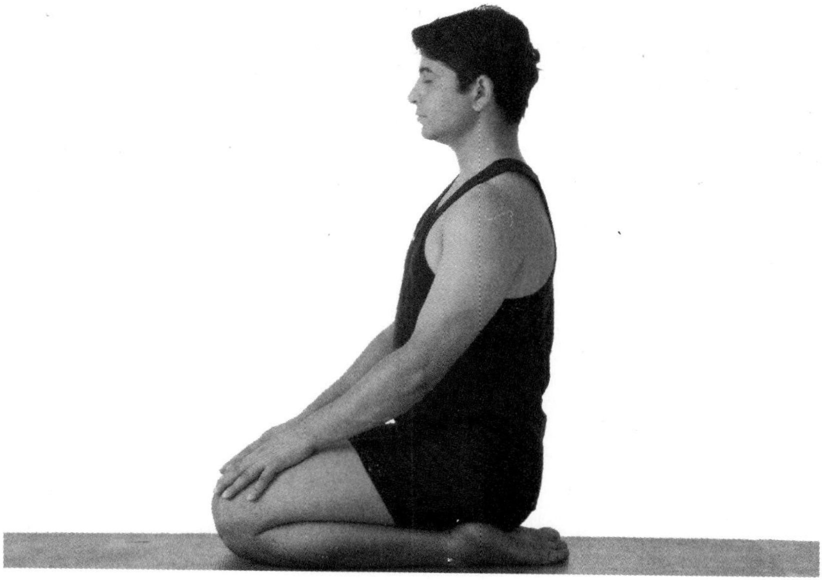

Kapalbhati Kriya

- Sit in *vajrasana* and close your eyes, keeping your back straight and your hands on your knees. Exhale forcefully from the nose and allow your stomach to move inwards. Allow the inhalations to happen automatically and focus only on the exhalations. Starting slowly, increase your speed, maintaining a rhythm. Start with 50 exhalations and increase to 100. Then relax for some time with your eyes closed.

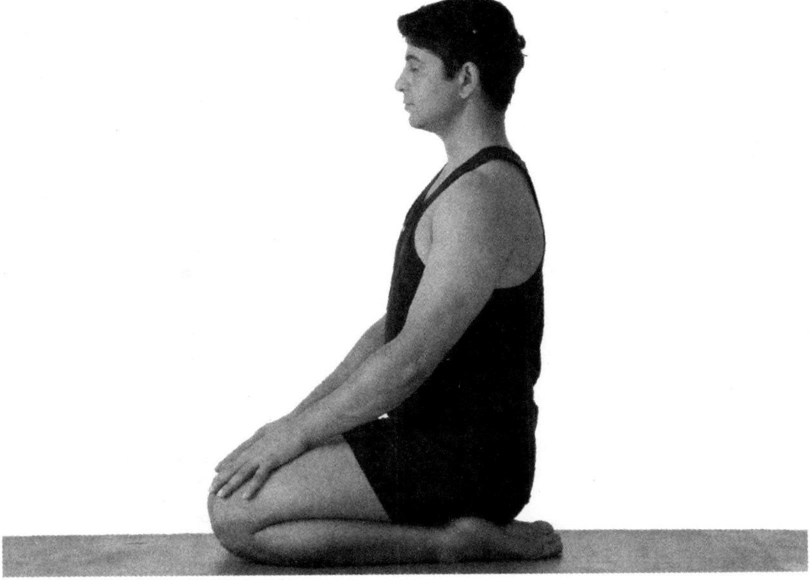